INTERMITTENT FASTING FOR WOMEN

First edition. August 18, 2018.

ISBN: 978-1727053722

Written by Christine Bailey.

Intermittent Fasting For Women

Powerful Strategies To Burn Fat & Lose Weight Rapidly, Control Hunger, Slow The Aging Process, & Live A Healthy Life As You Keep Your Hormones In Balance

Introduction

I AM SO GLAD YOU TOOK time out of your busy schedule to purchase your copy of *Intermittent Fasting for Women*. Thank you for doing so!

The following chapters will provide you with all the necessary information about this subject, such as how intermittent fasting isn't a new fad at all—it has been around for a very long time. This book explains intermittent fasting techniques in detail so you can see your choices regarding your plan to fast and lose those extra pounds. Each of the recipes in this book will address your program using the ketogenic low-carb dieting plan. But wait; it is also so much more than that. It can provide you with so many other health benefits.

Intermittent fasting has grown in popularity in recent years, thanks in large part to its ability to promote higher rates of nutrient absorption in the meals you eat. It has also grown in popularity because it doesn't require that its followers radically change the types of foods they eat and the times of day when they consume those foods. It doesn't even call for a drastic alteration of the number of calories a person consumes in each 24-hour period. In fact, the most common type of intermittent fasting is to simply eat two slightly larger-than-average meals during the day instead of the usual three.

This makes the intermittent fasting diet plan an ideal choice for those who have trouble sticking to more stringent diet plans, as it requires changing only one habit—number of meals per day—instead of many habits all at once. Many people find that intermittent fasting leads to real results. It's simple enough to manage successfully over a prolonged period, and efficient enough to provide the type of results that can maintain motivation even after the novelty begins to fade.

The secret to intermittent fasting's success is the simple fact that your body behaves differently in a fasting state than it does in a fed state. When your body is in what is known as a fed state, it is actively digesting and absorbing food. This begins some five minutes after you have finished putting food into your body and can last anywhere from three to five hours, depending on how difficult the food is for your body to digest. While in the fed state, your body is actively producing insulin, which makes the body less capable of properly burning fat.

During the period after digestion, insulin levels start dropping back to normal, which can take anywhere from eight to 12 hours. This is the buffer between the fed and fasting states. Once your insulin levels return to normal, the fasting state begins. This is the period when your body can process fat most effectively. Unfortunately, as people rarely go eight hours, much less 12 hours, without some type of caloric consumption, this means that many people never reach a point at which they can burn fat efficiently.

There is hope! *However*, to start seeing real results, you'll need to break the three-meals-a-day habit.

Follow the Golden Rules of Intermittent Fasting as provided in this informative book. In each segment, you will also discover many new tips and fresh guidelines. In the end, you will know how to prepare healthier meals while on the fasting protocol, using the great recipes included in the later chapters. For each of your meals, you can use your Instant Pot, Crock-Pot, stovetop, oven, or other food appliance to prepare healthy breakfast, lunch, and dinnertime meals. As you will soon see, this undertaking is not as hard as you think!

Plenty of books about this subject are available on the market, so thanks again for choosing this one! Every effort was made to ensure that it is full of as much useful information as possible. Please enjoy each topic to its fullest!

Chapter 1: Intermittent Fasting as a Woman

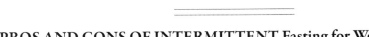

PROS AND CONS OF INTERMITTENT Fasting for Women

Even with all the benefits of the intermittent fasting technique, it is unfortunate that women are naturally more sensitive to signals of starvation. This is how it happens. Once your body senses famine, courtesy of the hunger hormones leptin and ghrelin, it prompts the feeling of hunger.

Leptin is the active hormone that controls the appetite. It gives the signal to stop eating when the body has reached its "full" state. Once your fast begins, your body stops producing as much leptin. Ghrelin is the hormone that prompts the "hunger" mode. Fasting triggers the production of ghrelin, making its levels rise dramatically. You get hungry, and the cravings begin. It also slows the metabolism rate.

This hormone imbalance can disrupt your hormones and lead to the following issues:

- Depression and anxiety
- Shrinking ovaries
- Difficulty sleeping
- Fertility issues
- Irregular or missed period (amenorrhea) caused by a lack of leptin in your system
- Headaches caused by a drop in blood glucose levels (hypoglycemia) during fasting

You can reduce these problems by choosing the right method. Following are some of the important points to consider before choosing your plan:

- The ideal fast is 12-16 hours.

- It is highly inadvisable to fast for over 24 hours at a time.
- Drink plenty of fluids during your fast.
- During your first two to three weeks of fasting, don't fast on consecutive days. For example, choose to fast for three days instead of seven.
- On your fasting days, do only light exercises, including gentle stretching, walking, jogging, or yoga.

Is Intermittent Fasting Suitable for You?

Ask yourself these questions to discover whether any of the intermittent plans will help you:

- Do I want to become pregnant?
- Am I pregnant?
- Have I ever suffered from eating disorders such as anorexia?
- Do I have diabetes?
- Do I have hypoglycemia?
- Am I underweight?

Clue: If you answered "no" to each question, you are a suitable candidate for the diet technique. If you said "yes" to any or all of them, it is definitely not the time for you to start this program.

Following are additional indications that intermittent fasting is not ideal for you.

Type 1 diabetics: Your blood sugar naturally drops when you fast. If you are on insulin-lowering drugs, you will need to consult your physician before you begin the fasting process. It is possible for you to lower the dosage during your dieting.

Thyroid and adrenal issues: Proceed with caution because individuals with either of these problems have issues dealing with stress. Fasting has been perceived as exacerbating this pre-existing condition.

Children: Until a child reaches his/her 18th birthday, fasting is not advisable. Children are still growing and require more nutrients daily.

When Women Should Avoid Intermittent Fasting

As a woman, you have additional stress factors, including times when the special fasting techniques are not a good fit for you. Here are a few:

- When you're nursing

- When you're pregnant
- When you're under chronic stress
- When you have difficulty sleeping or have sleep disorders
- When you have had a previous food disorder such as anorexia or bulimia

Fasting and Your Hormones

Put simply, your body experiences insatiable hunger if you start undereating. The female body would react as if it were protecting a "potential" fetus—even if you aren't pregnant. Many women ignore the hunger "cues" and binge later. However, the vicious cycle of undereating can halt ovulation and send your hormones out of whack.

The theory of intermittent fasting was tested for two weeks using female rats. The female indeed stopped having a menstrual cycle, and the ovaries shrank. Females experienced more instances of insomnia than did their male counterparts. However, the males did produce less testosterone. Though few human studies have been performed that reflect the same scientific understanding, the issues are still there.

Intermittent Fasting and Post-Menopause

Are you one of those women who worries about gaining belly fat and increased body weight after menopause? If you are, you have the tools at hand to keep those extra bulges under control. Not only that, intermittent fasting doesn't have an adverse effect on your bones during the aging process. So ladies, chin up and enjoy the fasting techniques this diet plan uses during intermittent fasting.

Benefits of Intermittent Fasting

Other than weight loss, you can benefit from intermittent fasting in many ways. You will live a longer life by achieving an extended fasting state and diverting your energy while improving your biological functions.

Just remember, the plan will not in any way cause you to starve. The emergency signals that your body sends out are simply that—signals. The fasting state your body experiences will diminish once your body adjusts to the method of intermittent fasting you choose to implement.

These are some of the crucial elements to consider:

Anti-aging: While the process has been tested using only animals, the rats tested lived 36% to 83% longer than did those that did not undergo fasting.

Heart health: This plan can reduce blood triglycerides, LDL cholesterol, insulin resistance, and blood sugar. Each of these presents a considerable risk element for heart ailments or disease.

Brain health: Your brain hormone BDNF—also known as brain-derived "neurotropic" factor—is a protein that can promote the growth of new nerve cells. Fasting is also believed to provide protection against Alzheimer's and Parkinson's diseases.

Cancer: Studies using animals have suggested that intermittent fasting can help prevent the disease.

Insulin resistance: Your blood sugar levels can be lowered by 3.0 to 3.6%, while fasting insulin levels can decrease by as much as 20 to 31%. These figures indicate that you should be better protected against type 2 diabetes, as well as have a more stable level of mood and energy stages.

Inflammation: Chronic diseases are driven by inflammation. Fasting plans using ketogenic diet methods help reduce swelling, as proven by private studies. Your body can repair itself, heal, and recover more quickly than it could without the diet plan.

Fatty acid oxidation: With the oxidation process, your body will burn more fats as energy. This will also provide for quick weight loss.

Lower stress levels: Cortisol production is lowered.

Note: Each of these studies is in its early stages. More research must be done using human testing during the fasting process.

Scientific Proof: The Plan Works

Because of hormonal changes, short-term fasting increases your metabolic rate from 3.6 to 14%. Studies have established that weight loss after three to 24 weeks on the intermittent fasting program can be maintained at 3.0 to 8.0%. In comparison to other studies on weight loss, these are high percentages that cannot be ignored.

In the same studies, many of the individuals lost 4.0 to 7.0% of their waist circumference. This indicates how the harmful buildup of belly fat can cause disease and other issues around your organs. You must consider that these results stem from eating fewer overall calories, not from binging during days off. You must maintain a sensible eating program.

Follow the Guidelines: The Golden Rules

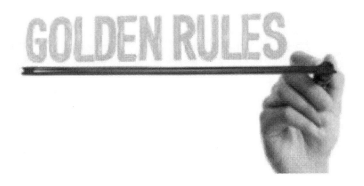

SCIENCE PROVIDES SPECIFIC proof that intermittent fasting is promising. When you start any new dietary plan, you will need to keep a few things in mind. No diet, regardless of how miraculous it appears, can help you if you don't obey a few golden rules.

Maintain your self-control: Intermittent fasting works only if your body goes entirely without food for at least 12 hours. Any caloric intake within that time resets the cycle. As such, it is imperative that you maintain control of your bodily urges if you hope to see real results from this type of approach. Remember, fasting for at least 12 hours will allow you to eat only as you usually would, or slightly more than an average meal. It does not give you license to eat everything in sight. Keeping your appetite in check is a strict requirement for success.

Remain consistent during fasting: Regardless of the type of weight loss you ultimately choose to pursue, you must pick one and stick with it. Attempting an intermittent fast for a few days before switching to another plan such as the Paleo diet, and then trying out a low-carb approach, will only cause your body to freak out. Your body will hold onto every possible calorie until it figures out what in the world is happening.

Remember, fasting regularly and consistently is the surest way to see any benefits. Only after your body has had time to adjust to your new routine will it be able to adapt appropriately. Using this method, it can begin increasing the number of positive enzymes and neural pathways to maximize weight loss. Consider consistency to be the "ace in the hole" of proactive weight loss success.

Maintain a calorie deficit: While this is true for any diet, it is even truer for intermittent fasting. Overeating after breaking your fast can be so easy. However, it negates any of the benefits you might otherwise have enjoyed. Remember, on average, you must burn 3,500 calories weekly to lose one pound each week.

Possible Side Effects

While intermittent fasting has some scientifically proven benefits, it is not without potential side effects.

Bowel issues: The biggest side effect is the initial change in your bowel movements, wherein periods of constipation or, in some cases, diarrhea could occur. Fortunately, they should not last more than a few days as your body adjusts to the new method of caloric intake.

Additional damage can be done to the body if you follow periods of fasting with periods of excessive binging. It is vital that you attempt intermittent fasting (and your periods of eating after) in moderation. If you notice immediate severe physical changes after you begin any form of dieting regime, you must consult a nutritionist or your physician.

Chapter 2: History, Alternatives, & How It Works

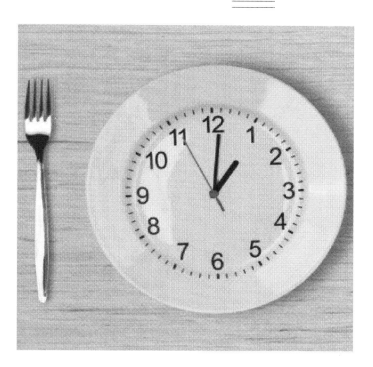

HISTORY OF INTERMITTENT Fasting

Fasting is not a recent trend. It has been part of some religious beliefs, including Buddhism, Islam, and Christianity, for centuries. Decades before this generation, the process may have been brought on by the unavailability of food resources. However, bear in mind that it is not a starvation diet because starvation is considered an involuntary absence of food. Consider breakfast to be the most crucial time of your day. After all, it is called such because it is when you "break" your "fast"—a natural part of anyone's day.

Fasting as we know it dates back to Hippocrates of Cos (c. 460–c370 BC), whom many consider to be the father of modern medicine. He stated, "To eat when you are sick is to feed your illness." Plato, an ancient Greek thinker, and

Aristotle, his student, believed in and supported fasting. The Greeks believed that fasting was the "physician within." This is the same logic and instinct that your pets maintain.

Benjamin Franklin, a prominent founding father of America, also stated, "The best of all medicine is resting and fasting."

Our American Diet Has Failed

Americans, on average, consume nearly 2,600 calories daily. That total is approximately 500 calories more than what Americans consumed 40 years ago, according to the USDA. Since the 1970s, over 92% of the uptick can be attributed to grains, fats, and oils.

Do the math. Thirty years ago, the combination was roughly 37% of our daily calories. The boost in fast food consumption has increased the amount of processed foods we consume in our regular diet plans. A 2013 study by the USDA's Economic Research Service confirmed the statistics: Fast food accounted for 3% of the US diet in 1977 and 1978. Between 2005 and 2008, it had jumped up to 13%.

According to the American Journal of Clinical Nutrition (2007), over the last 160 years, sugar intake has been on the rise, with people in Western countries, consuming about 150 pounds yearly. The total can be equated to an excess of 500 calories from sugar daily, which is more than our bodies can handle. The sugar continues to cause diseases, such as type 2 diabetes, obesity, cancer, and heart disease. Consumption of fruit juice and sodas has also experienced a huge increase. One study with children indicated a 60% increased risk of obesity.

These calories are attacking Americans' waistlines. Individuals 20 and older are now three times more likely to become obese than were individuals 30 years ago. According to The Washington Post, those tallies indicate that the USA is the "most obese" major country in the world. The aftermath is an economic problem as well. According to the CDC, in recent years almost $150 billion was spent on treatment of obesity.

You may well ask, how did this happen? Many individuals replaced heart-healthy butter with trans-fat-laden margarine, traditionally made with hydrogenated oils. By consuming grass-fed butter, you can fight heart disease with vitamin K12. In 1999, soybean oil provided 7% of the calories in the American diet. The source is usually added to processed foods because it is cheap.

Take a stand and choose to change these statistics! If you are asking how you can do this, know that you already began the journey when you purchased your new intermittent fasting book. The recipes the book provides will use a special low-carb diet plan called the ketogenic diet. The next section will describe how the plan works by using your calories, carbohydrates, and proteins to keep your body in a state of ketosis for weight loss.

The Role of Calories, Protein, and Carbs

To achieve weight loss, you will need to reduce your carbohydrate intake and achieve ketosis. You will soon realize that, by using the ketogenic diet plan in this book, you can feel full and satisfied while still losing weight. You simply need to restrict your carb intake, including starches such as bread and pasta, as well as sugars. Following the keto diet, you will replace these unwanted elements with fat and protein. Not only will you lose weight, you will lower your blood pressure, triglycerides, and blood sugar.

What works for one person as a low-carb diet may be insufficient for another person. It depends on your activity levels, age, body composition, and gender. It may also depend on your metabolic health, food culture, and personal preferences. If you are more active and have more muscle mass, you can tolerate more carbs than can someone who is sedentary. If people get metabolic syndrome, they may become obese or suffer from type 2 diabetes. As such, the rules would change. Scientists sometimes refer to this condition as carbohydrate intolerance.

As mentioned, there's no set rule for carb intake. Following are some of the basic guidelines to consider as you blaze a path towards the ketogenic diet plan, which is effective about 90% of the time:

20-50 grams daily: Losing weight at the rate of 20-50 grams daily falls into this category. If you have diabetes, are obese, or are metabolically deranged, this is the plan for you. If you are consuming less than 50 grams daily, your body will achieve a ketosis state that supplies the ketone bodies.

Consider these guidelines:

- Plenty of low-carbohydrate veggies
- Some berries with whipped cream
- Trace carbs from foods including nuts, seeds, and avocados

50-100 grams daily:

- Plenty of veggies
- Two or three pieces of fruit every day
- Minimal intake of starchy carbs

Moderate carb intake—100-150 grams daily: If you are active and lean and are trying to maintain weight, these are some foods to consider:

- All the veggies you can eat
- Several fruits daily
- Healthy starches such as rice, oats, sweet potatoes, and potatoes

As you can see, before you make any changes, it is important to experiment and categorize where you fall on the scales. Seek your doctor's advice before you change your eating patterns. In this way, you will achieve ketosis, which is also a goal using the intermittent fasting methods that the enclosed guidelines describe.

How the Keto Plan Works

A ketogenic diet will help you reduce your calorie intake to below the volume of calories your body can expend in one day. Therefore, you must summon the energy stored in your fat cells to deliver fuel/energy to your muscles.

The keto diet will limit the volume of carbs you consume. A substantial portion of your daily fuel will come from fat content, which is converted to ketones. You can achieve a great deal of fat burning on a greater amount of calories by sustaining food options that the ketogenic plan uses. When you maintain the protein, carbohydrates, and fat ratio monitored by the diet plan, as shown in this cookbook, you will be well on your way to a successful diet strategy.

You will not be overeating with large portions of protein. You won't eliminate fat or carbs. This makes it a useful and safe diet plan for fat loss. If you take the approach of eating less without considering your diet, you will lose the essential minerals and vitamins that you need daily. This could result in muscle spasms, fatigue, mental fogginess, hunger, headaches, irritability, insomnia, and emotional depression. You could also lose valuable muscle mass, not just the pounds you intended to drop.

By using the lower carb keto plan, you can reduce your carbohydrates and calorie counts, as well as nurture your body with the suitable amount of water, meat, eggs, fish, veggies, nuts, and high-quality oils that create fat loss minus the unpleasant side effects.

The Process

Ketosis helps you drop extra pounds and burn body fat using healthy eating practices. Proteins will fuel your body to burn the fat. In turn, ketosis will maintain your muscles and make you less hungry.

Your body will remain healthy and will work as it should. If you don't consume enough carbs from your food, your cells will instead burn fat for the necessary energy. Your body will switch over to ketosis for its energy source as you cut back on your calories and carbs.

Elements of Ketosis: Lipogenesis and Glycogenesis

Two stages occur when your body doesn't need glucose:

- **The stage of lipogenesis:** If your liver and muscles have a sufficient supply of glycogen, any excess is converted into fat and stored.

- **The stage of glycogenesis:** The excess glucose is converted into glycogen and stored in the muscles and liver. Research indicates that only about half the energy you use daily can be saved as glycogen.

When the glycerol and fatty acid molecules are released, the ketogenesis process begins, and acetoacetate is produced. The acetoacetate is converted into two types of ketone units:

- **Acetone:** This is mostly excreted as waste, but it can also be metabolized into glucose. This is the reason why individuals on a ketogenic diet experience a distinctive smelly breath.

- **Beta-hydroxybutyrate or BHB:** Your muscles will convert the acetoacetate into BHB, which will fuel your brain after you have been on the keto diet for a short time.

Your body will lack food (similar to when you are sleeping), making your body burn the stored fat to create ketones. Once the ketones break down the fats, which generate fatty acids, they will burn off in the liver through beta-oxidation. Thus, when you no longer have a supply of glycogen or glucose, ketosis begins and will use the consumed/stored fat as energy.

A keto calculator can be found at "keto-calculator.ankerl.com." You can check your levels when you want to know which nutrients your body needs during your dieting plan or afterward. Document your personal information, such as height and weight. The calculator will provide you with the essential math.

Powerful Alternatives Using Intermittent Fasting

The specifics of when you fast are not nearly as important as ensuring that you fast for the same period of time as regularly as possible. If you vary your fasting period too much, the result can be an erratic change in your hormones, which, among other things, makes it much more difficult for your body to shed excess weight. If you find yourself without time to eat a proper meal to break your fast, ensure that you eat at least something to keep your body on the correct cycle.

While the core ideas behind the various forms of intermittent fasting are similar, there are many different ways to go about them. Your best bet is to try a few and see which one your body naturally responds to the easiest. Just remember to not cut the calories too much at first. As an example, an average woman who usually consumes 1600 calories should consume approximately 530 calories on a fasting day.

Crescendo Method: Use this technique to dive into fasting without aggravating your hormones or shocking any part of your body. This is one of the safest programs for women. It utilizes a fasting window of 12-16 hours. You can enjoy your meals for eight to 12 hours. Space it out across a few days, e.g., Monday, Wednesday, and Friday. If you have failed other diets, this might be your answer. After a two-week time period, add one more day of active fasting to your schedule.

16/8 Method: This technique is often referred to as the "lean-gains method." Its routine explicitly targets your body fat and creates leaner muscle mass. One of the most significant benefits of this type of fasting is that it's incredibly flexible—it will work well if you have a varied schedule. This safe program provides a fasting window of 16 hours, with the hours of eating at eight.

This method involves fasting for 14 hours for women (compared to 16 hours for men) before consuming a reasonable quantity of calories for the remaining eight to 10 hours. Most people find it helpful to either eat two large meals during the eight- or 10-hour feeding period or to split that time into three smaller meals, as this is how most people are already programmed.

The Obesity Society performed a study stating that if you have your dinner before 2:00 p.m., your hunger yearnings will drop for the remainder of the day. At the same time, your fat-burning reserves will be boosted. During the fasting period, you should consume only items with zero calories, including black coffee (a splash of cream is excellent), water, diet soda, and sugar-free gum. The easiest way to attempt this schedule is to stop eating after dinner in the evening and wait 14 hours from there. This means skipping breakfast and picking things up in the early afternoon.

24-Hour Protocol: This technique is also known as the "Eat-Stop-Eat" technique. It requires that you do a 24-hour fast no more than twice a week. You can choose the time when you start fasting. Many believe it is easier to fast from 8 pm to 8 pm because so much of the time, you will be asleep. You automatically go into ketosis.

When you are done fasting, you must eat a reasonable or regular diet and avoid binging for an extended period. Fast/binge cycles can severely damage your body. As always, moderation and self-control are necessary to get the most out of the fasting cycle.

This fast cycle works on the assumption that to lose a pound of weight a week, you must give up 3,500 calories. It might be best to get it out of the way in two quick bursts rather by fasting for a portion of every single day. This fasting plan emphasizes resistance weight training for maximum benefits.

For some people, going a full day without eating can be difficult at first. However, it is perfectly doable to work up to a full day of fasting by holding out as long as possible and increasing that amount of time through practice. An excellent way to start is by choosing days when you don't have any prior food commitments. Beginning a fasting program on a day when you know you have a lunch meeting is a bad idea.

When you first start this fast cycle, fatigue, headaches, or feelings of anger or anxiousness are all common side effects. They should be considered good stopping points for your current fast. These side effects will diminish as your body adjusts to the new cycle.

After you go a full day without calories, you will naturally have the desire to binge during your first meal. You must have the self-control to fight these urges because not only is binging bad for you, it can also quickly undo all your hard work from the previous 24 hours. Practice self-discipline and make your fasting worth the effort.

The 5:2 Diet: The 5:2 diet, also known as the "Fast Diet," involves restricting calories two days a week to 500 calories per day (with two 250-calorie meals) while eating regularly for the other five days. Not many statistics are available about this diet for women, but it is considered safe. Choosing two days to fast and assuming your regular caloric intake for the remaining five days is an easy process.

The Warrior Diet: The Warrior Diet takes the 16:8 Program and kicks it up a notch by recommending that you fast for roughly 20 hours out of each day. This is followed by one meal that gives you all of your calories for the day's four remaining hours.

This form of intermittent fasting follows the belief that humans are naturally nocturnal eaters. Eating at night helps the body better process the nutrients it needs. In this case, fasting is a bit of a misnomer, as during the 20-hour period, you are allowed to eat a serving of raw vegetables or fruits, and maybe a serving of protein if you can't otherwise continue.

This works because it causes the body's natural sympathetic nervous system to activate a flight or fight response, which in turn increases your natural levels of alertness and energy while simultaneously increasing the amount of fat you burn. The large meal each evening allows the body to focus on repairing itself and improving its muscles. When you follow the Warrior Diet, you must start each evening meal with vegetables, then proceed to the protein, fat, and carbohydrates that the keto diet uses.

This form of fasting is well-known for two reasons. First, the fact that it allows a few small and reasonable snacks during the fasting process makes this type of fasting attractive to those who are attempting the practice for the first time. Second, nearly everyone who tries this form of fasting reports a significant amount of increased energy throughout the day as well as an increase in the amount of fat they lose per week.

On the other hand, this diet's relatively strict nature can make it difficult for some people to follow for long periods of time. The timing of the large meal can also be problematic for some people because it can naturally interfere with social engagements. Finally, some people don't like having to eat their food in a specific order. Try it for yourself and see what works for you.

Fat Loss Forever: This form of intermittent fasting combines elements of several other styles of fasting to create something unique. The good news is that you get a cheat day every week. The bad news is that this cheat day is followed by a one-and-a-half-day fast. The remainder of the week is split between 16:8 and 20:4 fasting.

For this diet, you must schedule your exercise rest days for the second part of the 36-hour cycle. Otherwise, you must stay as busy as possible on these days to help combat your hunger. If you have trouble controlling your appetite on cheat days, this form of intermittent fasting may not be for you, as it requires that you go from 60 to zero quickly and regularly.

Also, it is important to not go 36 hours without eating food all at once. You will need to build up your body's tolerance for fasting. As such, it is usually better to start with another form of intermittent fasting. Work up to the Fat Loss Forever method after your body has already gotten out of the habit of eating every three or four hours.

Always remember to fast responsibly, and never push your body to the point that you feel physically ill. Also, remember to fast following a routine to give your body the time it needs to adjust to the change.

Alternate Day Diet: This form of intermittent fasting means you never have to go long without food if you so choose. Every other day, you should eat regularly. On the off-days, you simply consume one-fifth of the calories you intake on the average days.

The average daily caloric consumption is between 2,000 and 2,500 calories, which means the regular off-day varies between 400 and 500 calories. If you enjoy exercising every day, this form of intermittent fasting may not be for you, as you will have to greatly curtail your workouts on off-days.

When you first start this form of intermittent fasting, the easiest way to make it through the low-calorie days is to try any one of a variety of protein shakes. It is important to work back to "real" natural foods on these days because they will always be healthier than the shakes.

This form of intermittent fasting is all about losing weight. Those who try it tend to average between two and three pounds lost per week. If you attempt the Alternate Day Diet, you must eat regularly on your full-calorie days. Binging will not only negate any progress you have made, but also severely damage your body if you continue doing so over time.

IRREGULARLY SKIPPING Meals

If you are interested in experiencing the benefits of intermittent fasting for yourself but have an irregular schedule or aren't sure whether it's for you, skipping a meal or two now and then might be the type of intermittent fasting that is most suitable for you. As previously discussed, getting into a fasting routine is vital to see maximum results for your effort. However, occasionally, that also means fasting doesn't come with some benefits.

What's more, once you have tried skipping a meal now and then, you can see for yourself just how easy it is. This, in turn, can lead to more positive changes down the road. With so many intermittent fasting options available, the odds are good that one will fit your schedule, so give it a try. What do you have to lose (besides a few pounds)?

Chapter 3: Make the Process Work

EXERCISE AND INTERMITTENT Fasting

If you are exercising as well as intermittently fasting, you must ensure that while you are working out, you are eating more carbohydrates than fats. On days when you are not exercising, the opposite should be true. Keep your protein intake at a steady level. Stay away from processed foods whenever possible.

On days when you are exercising as well as fasting, you must break your fast with a mix of protein, vegetables, and fruit. If you generally go to the gym directly after you have broken your fast, you must include enough carbohydrates to give your muscles the energy they need to get the most out of your workout.

If you are planning to exercise, it is usually best to start your early afternoon on a healthy note with a medium-calorie meal. Then, you must exercise either within three hours, before eating a more substantial meal, or soon afterward. For this more critical meal, you must add an increased portion of complex carbohydrates. You can even have a little dessert as long as it is in moderation. Remember, fasting is different from dieting.

On days when you do not plan to exercise, you must adjust your caloric intake appropriately. Start by limiting your carbohydrate intake. Focus instead on eating lots of protein, dark green, leafy vegetables, and fruit in moderation. Unlike on days when you are exercising, the first meal you eat on rest days should be your largest in terms of caloric intake. This one meal should account for about 40% of your daily total.

Remember, during this meal, you should take in more protein than anything else. For your final dinner during rest days, include a protein source that will take lots of time to digest. This means it will keep you full for much of your fast the following morning. It will also give the body enough stored amino acids to prevent it from breaking down muscle during the fast.

Tips & Tricks

While intermittent fasting is undeniably beneficial, it can be challenging to get started or to see it through to the point at which your body adapts to a new schedule. The following tips and tricks can set you on the path to success.

Pay attention to your body talk: While you must keep tabs on how your body is responding to intermittent fasting, it is doubly important to monitor your vitals during the initial phase, when your body is adjusting to the new feeding times. Expect some discomfort for the first three to four weeks. However, anything longer or more severe than that should be discussed with a doctor as soon as possible.

Be sure the plan is for you: Intermittent fasting offers a wide variety of proven benefits, but it is not for everyone. Before you attempt a fast, have a real dialogue with yourself. Consider your level of self-discipline, your current attachment to food, regular activities that would make fasting difficult or awkward, your general lifestyle, and your level of exercise. Deciding to try a different fitness regime is a lot easier on day one than it is after struggling through a week or more of faulty fasting.

Set lower goals; start slowly: If you are having trouble starting the transition to an intermittent fasting program, try moving your breakfast time back one hour each week. Before you know it, you will have reached a 16:8 or 14:10 split without even trying.

Keep it a secret: While plenty of scientific evidence supports intermittent fasting, skeptics are still out there. You don't need that negativity, especially when you are first starting out. After you have started seeing results, you will more easily be able to defend the process to non-believers. Just show them a before-and-after picture.

No excuses: Intermittent fasting works on the principle that eating fewer calories than you burn is a surefire way to lose weight. This theory falls apart if you use the fact that you are fasting as an excuse to eat nothing but junk food when the time comes to break your fast. Self-control and self-discipline are both equally important when it comes to eating correctly. Intermittent fasting has a wide variety of health benefits. Why not accentuate them even more with a healthy diet?

Begin your day hydrated: Often, the signals for hunger and the signs of thirst get crossed in your brain. After it has sent out enough ignored thirst signals, the brain starts sending out hunger signals instead. As such, starting the morning by drinking at least half a liter of water is an excellent way to quench your body's thirst after the past seven or eight hours. This should be enough to keep you feeling full for at least a few extra hours each morning. Not only will water help you feel full throughout your fast, but staying hydrated is akin to staying healthy. Aim for at least a gallon of water per day.

Caffeine can naturally suppress your appetite: Black coffee works best, as there is little in it that can negatively affect your metabolism or general wellbeing. The same cannot be said for most zero-calorie caffeinated beverages. Artificial sweeteners have been shown to cause some health problems. Still, anything with caffeine will help calm your appetite for at least a little while.

Ups and downs: While your body adjusts to intermittent fasting, there will be times when you are losing weight and times when your body is trying to hold on to every calorie it has. This is natural and to be expected as your body realigns its hormone levels.

When you're hungry: Consider the difference between head hunger and body hunger. As you get used to the process of intermittent fasting, you will become familiar with several different types of hunger. Ultimately, you will learn how to determine when you are "truly" hungry as opposed to habitually accustomed to eating. While telling the difference will be difficult initially, you will come to know them both intimately in time.

Get off to the right start "fast": At the start of your fast, your body will still have the most fuel in its system to work with. This is why it is best to start each fast with the most challenging items on your to-do list. As you move further from the last period of time and take in fresh calories, your thought processes will naturally slow due to your body's effort to save energy. Difficult tasks will seem more natural when your body is working at maximum efficiency.

Be patient for the best results: As previously discussed, your body will need time to fully adjust to your new dietary patterns and to start reflecting these new results. Try intermittent fasting regularly for at least a month before rendering judgment about the plan's success.

Shuffle your schedule: After you have given your body time to adjust to an intermittent fasting schedule, take the time to fluctuate your on/off patterns throughout the day to see what works best for you. Taking the time to experiment may yield unexpected results.

Make the fasting time work for you: Intermittent fasting can work around any type of schedule. This is part of what makes it so great. If you find yourself feeling trapped by the period of time during which you allow yourself to eat, why not adjust it? Fasting should be about adding freedom to your schedule, not restraining it.

Stay busy: Don't spend the latter parts of your fast simply waiting to eat. Intermittent fasting can be either extremely difficult or surprisingly easy depending solely on the amount of time you spend thinking about food. Find ways to occupy your mind and you will be surprised by how quickly meal time rolls around.

Consume sufficient amounts of protein: Nothing is better at combating hunger than protein, plain and simple. It is also great for building lean muscle. If you find yourself unable to get through even 10 hours without eating, this might be a sign that you should add more protein to your diet.

Try branched-chain amino acids: For those on a low-calorie diet such as intermittent fasting, studies show that a BCAA supplement stimulates additional fat loss while simultaneously preventing lean muscle from being consumed as the body tries to feed itself.

Go slow—not fast: Even if you think you feel okay when you first begin an intermittent fasting cycle, it is crucial to give your body the time it needs to recover. Never go more than two days out of a week without eating. There is an essential distinction between fasting and starving yourself.

Distract yourself: Distraction is necessary while your body is adapting to your new eating habits. It becomes increasingly important the further into a fast you get. When you are struggling with the plan, being active can help you refocus your thinking patterns. The exercise can also push away the pounds.

How to break your fast: The content and quality of your first meal of the day can quickly set the tone for those that follow. Use this to your advantage by starting your feeding window with something healthy. You will be surprised at how much this improves your willpower for later meals.

Don't use fasting to hide from other issues: Those with a tendency to develop eating disorders or those who believe they might have one should stay away from intermittent fasting, as it can quickly lead to more pressing issues if not appropriately controlled. Remember, while you must have the willpower to stop eating for a set period of time, it is equally important to have the willpower to begin eating again once the fast is over.

Perform moderate exercise: Dieting works by ensuring that you are taking in fewer calories than you are burning in a fixed period of time. As such, if you are trying one of the intermittent fasting options that involve not eating for a day or more, you must adjust your exercise plan for these days as well. When you exercise, your body requires fuel. If you don't give it another choice, it will take this fuel from your muscles. Over-exercising can become too much when you're fasting and is a sure-fire recipe for disaster.

Once again, listen to your body: Learn what your body is saying. Many people consider a sudden craving for a particular food to be an indication that they are hungry. They take action and respond accordingly. However, this craving is often brought on by an ancient part of the brain that believes salty, sweet, and high-fat foods are vital parts of a regular diet. Once upon a time, those three qualities equated to foods that were high in positive nutrients. This is no longer the case. In fact, it's the complete opposite. As such, you can safely ignore these urges. Take the time to investigate a sudden surge of hunger to see if it could actually be related to your emotional state instead of your physical one.

If you have followed the guidelines and are still not losing weight, you may need to consider other reasons. Ask yourself these questions:

Have I set unrealistic expectations?

Dropping pounds takes time. For most people, one to two pounds each week is sufficient; anything over that can become difficult to sustain all year long. If you were wrapped around junk food, your body is not conditioned to lose a massive amount of weight quickly. Recognize the potential amount you can reasonably lose over time.

Am I following the guidelines for a low-carb diet plan?

If you are not coupling yourself with the right action plan for fasting, you may not be sufficiently lowering your carbohydrate intake. Each of the recipes that this book provides will get you through the rough spots. Follow the ketogenic-style diet as described in your new cookbook. Maintain an intake of 20 to 50 grams of carbs daily. As a reference point, most individuals on a traditional diet consume 100 to 150 grams of carbs daily. Each of the provided recipes will guide you towards lowering the carb limits.

Am I counting macronutrients correctly?

Keep your nutrients in line. For the plan you are using (ketogenic), you will have a balanced ratio of fats, proteins, and carbs. Your body must remain in a ketosis state to achieve the desired results.

Do I have underlying health issues?

This cannot be stressed enough! Medications could affect your fasting needs. Check the side effects of your current medications and seek the advice of a qualified physician or nutritionist. If you are eating a wholesome, healthy diet as this plan describes but are seeing little results, you might have an undiagnosed medical problem. Set up an appointment for a checkup and get a blood test to rule out hidden medical issues.

Chapter 4: Maintain a Healthy Diet Plan

TO ADOPT A REALISTIC diet plan and maintain a new, desirable weight, you must understand your daily calorie needs. If the recipe does not indicate the calories, an adult BMI and Calorie Calculator[1] will be an essential tool. Most products you purchase will have ingredient panels listing the counts. Therefore, you will have a general idea of how to work your menu around your intermittent fasting plan.

You will need to enter your sex, height, weight, and age into the calculator. You will also need to give the calculator your daily activity schedule (such as daily, more than an hour, less than an hour, or rarely). The calculator will indicate your BMI score and the number of calories necessary to maintain your current body weight. It will make your goals easier to map by providing you with the tallies from your calculations to lower your counts.

The "No-No" Foods

After all the talk about the importance of natural foods, we'll now address some products to avoid so that your intermittent fast will be more effective. As a general rule, you should avoid the following foods, or at least limit them as much as possible.

Farm-raised salmon: Much like processed meat, farm-raised salmon is the least healthy type of an otherwise healthy meal choice. When salmon are raised in tubs near one another for prolonged periods of time, they lose much of their natural vitamin D and pick up traces of PCB, DDT, carcinogens, and bromine. Choose wild-caught fish if possible.

Processed meats: While protein is an undeniably important part of a healthy diet, seeking your protein from treated meats will stuff your body so full of chemicals that any benefits the meat might have had may end up lost. Compared to the quality of the cuts of meat found in most grocery stores, processed meats

---

1. https://www.bcm.edu/cnrc-apps/caloriesneed.cfm

tend to be lower in protein and higher in sodium and preservatives. This can cause a variety of health risks, including asthma and heart disease.

Non-organic milk: Despite being touted as part of a balanced diet, non-organic milk is routinely found to be full of growth hormones as well as puss as a result of the over-milking of cows. The growth hormones leave behind antibiotics which can, in turn, make it more difficult for the human body to counter infections. It can also cause an increased chance of colon cancer, prostate cancer, and breast cancer.

Non-organic potatoes: While starch and carbohydrates are vital parts of a balanced meal, non-organic potatoes are not worth the trouble. While still in the ground, they are treated with chemicals. Before they head to the store, they are treated again to ensure they stay "fresh" as long as possible. These chemicals have been shown to increase the risk of health issues like autism, asthma, birth defects, learning disabilities, Parkinson's and Alzheimer's diseases, and multiple types of cancer.

White flour: Much like processed meats, by the time white flour is done being processed, it is devoid of any nutritional value. When eaten as part of a regular diet, white flour has been shown to increase a woman's chance of suffering from breast cancer by a shocking 200%.

These are just a few of the reasons why processed foods should be considered a problem in the modern world. Processed foods can be regarded as any items containing preservatives, artificial colors, flavorings, additives, or chemicals that change the foods' texture. An additional significant warning sign of an unhealthy food is when it includes a substantial number of carbohydrates in its refined form.

In essence, the sooner you start taking the time to read labels and check ingredients, the sooner you can get the most out of the meals you eat in between intermittent fasting sessions. Making a conscious effort to do so may very well be the difference between life and death.

The "Yes" Foods

The components of a healthier eating pattern using intermittent fasting methods will account for all the beverages and foods on a suitable calorie level. A good plan for a healthy fasting pattern will include the following:

- Whole fruits
- Oils
- Grains (a minimum of half should be whole grains)
- Protein foods such as eggs, poultry, lean meats, seafood, nuts, seeds, and soy products
- Varied veggies from all the main subgroups, including starchy legumes (peas and beans), veggies colored red, orange, or dark green, and others

Health concerns in the USA focus on fundamental elements that should be limited when one follows the intermittent fasting diet plan. The recommendation is that you do the following:

- Consume less than 10% of your daily calories from saturated fats.
- Eat less than 10% of your daily intake of calories from added sugars.
- Maintain sodium consumption of less than 2,300 milligrams.
- Observe moderation if you consume alcohol products. Have no more than one each day if you are a woman and no more than two each day if you are a man.

Boost Your Metabolism:

Essential Minerals and Vitamins

Zinc, iron, and selenium are necessary for healthy bodily functions. Research has shown that a diet low in these elements reduces the thyroid gland's ability to produce vital hormones. This process will significantly slow metabolism. It is best to eat seeds, nuts, legumes, meat, and seafood. Enjoy some of these choices:

Pulses and legumes: This food group includes peanuts, lentils, chickpeas, beans, and peas, which are incredibly high in protein compared to other plant foods. According to research, the act of digesting higher protein counts requires the body to burn considerably more calories than it requires to digest lower protein foods. Recent studies have indicated that participants who consumed a legume-rich diet for eight weeks increased their metabolism rate and lost over 1.5 times more weight than did the control group.

Chili peppers: Chili peppers contain a chemical called capsaicin, which boosts metabolism. Capsaicin will increase the fat and calories you burn during your intermittent fasting plan. Twenty research studies have indicated that you would lose/burn approximately 50 extra calories daily. However, not all researchers agree with the theory.

Tea: Tea is considered a good beverage because of the catechins in the tea conglomerate, along with the caffeine that helps speed the metabolism. Catechins are an antioxidant and a type of natural phenol from the chemical family of flavonoids. The use of green and oolong tea can burn an additional 100 calories daily to increase your metabolism by 4 to 10%. The effects may be different for each individual.

Coffee: Your caffeine levels can help increase your metabolic rate by approximately 11%. Studies have shown that consumption of a minimum of 270 milligrams of caffeine—about three cups of coffee—will burn an additional 100 calories daily. The rates can surely boost your intermittent fasting as long as your coffee is sugar-free.

Protein-Rich Food Groups

Your body will need more energy to digest these products:

- Eggs
- Seeds and nuts
- Legumes
- Fish
- Meat

The thermic effect of food is referred to as TEF. This is the number of calories your body requires to absorb/digest the nutrients you receive in your meals. Protein intake will also give you a feeling of fullness that lasts much longer, possibly preventing you from overeating. Each of the following examples shows you how easy it is to convert to intermittent fasting if you choose the correct food groups.

The Good with the Bad

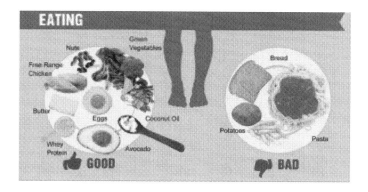

Examples of Good Food Groups

- Eggs and beans
- Seeds and nuts
- Eggs and potatoes
- Berries and whey protein
- Cocoa nibs and peanut butter

- Potatoes and peas
- Nuts and wine
- Cheese and wine
- Rice and beans

Examples of Poorly Chosen Food Groups

- Pasta and wine
- Pasta and nuts
- Raisins and nuts (trail mix)
- Sugar and cream
- Jelly and peanut butter
- Jam and bread
- Granola (honey nut)
- Sour foods

Chapter 5: Final Thoughts on Intermittent Fasting for Women

YOU HAVE NOW RECEIVED much of the information you need as a woman who wishes to try intermittent fasting. Remember to take it slow at first and make wise eating choices using your new recipes. If you slip, trust that you'll recover, and move on.

The ketogenic techniques work hand in hand with intermittent fasting for women. Here are a few pointers to get you going quickly:

Step 1: Choose the protocol you want to follow.

Step 2: Calculate the calories.

Step 3: Calculate the macronutrients.

Step 4: Create your personal meal plan.

You have plenty of meals to keep yourself busy for at least several weeks of fasting. There are also some quick and easy snacks to fill in the hunger spots. These won't cost you a lot of extra calories. For your convenience, the macronutrients for each of the recipes have been calculated. Follow the step-by-step instructions and you'll be on your way to a better mode of living.

Fasting Resources

Go online and contact a group called *Meetup* to find a support group that might be in your area. For example, these are just a few of the groups listed on the Internet:

- Fasting for Life | New York, NY
- Boston Fasting Solution | Somerville, MA[1]
- HVMN Intermittent Fasting Community[2] | San Francisco, CA[3]

---

1. https://www.meetup.com/cities/us/ma/somerville/

- Fasting Buddies[4] | London, ON[5]
- Keto Diet & Intermittent Fasting | Los Angeles, CA
- Supporting Keto & Intermittent Fasting | Conway, AR[6]

Ke

Another active resource is the Group Forum at the "Fat-Secret" website. There, you can discuss various topics starting from when you begin your journey. It is always helpful to share the ups and downs of your new experience with others who truly understand.

Lastly, get together with some of your friends and show the men how it's done!

Now, it's time to learn how to prepare your meals!

---

2. https://www.meetup.com/FastingMeetup/

3. https://www.meetup.com/cities/us/ca/san_francisco/

4. https://www.meetup.com/Fasting-Buddies/

5. https://www.meetup.com/cities/ca/on/london/

6. https://www.meetup.com/cities/us/ar/conway/

Chapter 6: Samples of "Grab & Go" Snacks

IF YOU ARE LIKE MANY people, when you hear the word "diet," you panic or assume that sticking to it will be difficult. This segment will acquaint you with some of the easiest and quickest techniques if you have a busy lifestyle. Snack time doesn't have to be boring. Add some of these healthier choices to your intermittent fasting meal plan for weight loss. Use a small plate to trick your mind into not overindulging. You will also notice how the "not-so-healthy" choices are those with higher calorie contents. One advantage of planning your menu before you are hungry is that you can avoid them.

Fruity Breakfast Meals

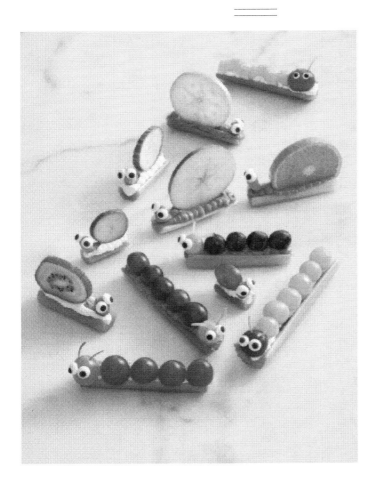

HONEY AND BANANAS

- 10 Calories: ½ tsp. honey
- 89 Calories: 1 small banana

Apricots and Yogurt

- 68 Calories: 2 chopped apricots and 25g Greek yogurt (low-fat)

Apricots, Greek Fat-Free Yogurt, and Mixed Berries

- 24 Calories: 3 tbsp. Greek yogurt
- 17 Calories: 1 apricot
- 19 Calories: 50g raspberries
- 16 Calories: 50g strawberries
- 20 Calories: 50g blackberries
- Total Calories: 96

Watermelon

- 96 Calories: 300g serving
- Note: Its natural sugars are more beneficial than a cereal bar.

Tasty Delights to Keep You Going Until Lunchtime

- 130 Calories: 1 square dark chocolate and a small banana
- 55 Calories: 10g of 85% dark chocolate
- 75 Calories: 3 stuffed celery sticks with low-fat cottage cheese
- 96 Calories: 16 olives (green or black)
- 90 Calories: 1 c. cherries
- 29 Calories: 100g honeydew melon
- 42 Calories: 2 satsumas/tangerine (The Christmas Orange)
- 90 Calories: 3 thin slices of pineapple
- 61 Calories: 100g grapes OR 100 Calories: 30 grapes
- 42 Calories: Sun-Maid mini box of raisins
- 90 Calories: 25 pistachio nuts
- 74 Calories: 10 salted peanuts

100-Calorie Items

- 31 asparagus spears
- 9 5-inch spears of broccoli
- 16 ribs of celery
- 12 raw Brussels sprouts
- 28 baby carrots
- 82 red kidney beans
- 60 raw green beans
- 43 boiled or steamed okra pods
- 100 radishes
- 20 sun-dried tomatoes
- 22 cloves of garlic
- 100 raspberries
- 5 dried figs
- 6 dried apricots
- 8 cashew nuts
- 10 Pringles chips
- 21 pretzels, unsalted minis
- 4 sardines in oil, drained
- 13 large boiled or steamed shrimp
- 15 pieces dry-roasted cashew halves

YOU CAN PREPARE THESE snacks in Ziploc baggies or similar containers. Grab a healthier treat and stay in line with your fasting calorie intake!

Chapter 7: Breakfast Delights

Beverages

Berry Mango Slush

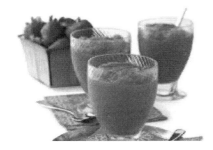

YIELDS: 4 SERVINGS (7.5 oz. each)

Nutrients: 5 net carbs ~ 0g protein ~ 0g fats ~ 20 cal.

Ingredients:

1 c. fresh strawberries

½ c. mango

1½ c. berry-flavored carbonated water, chilled

2 tsp. lime juice

How to prepare:

1. Slice the berries and chop the peeled mango.
2. Add all the fixings into a blender. Cover tightly and blend until slushy.
3. Serve right away in four chilled glasses.

Bulletproof Coffee

YIELDS: 1 SERVING

Nutrients: -0- net carbs ~ 1g protein ~ 51g fats ~ 463 cal.

Ingredients:

2 tbsp. MCT oil powder

2 tbsp. ghee/butter

1½ c. hot coffee

How to prepare:

1. Empty the hot coffee into a blender.
2. Pour in the powder and butter. Blend until frothy.
3. Enjoy in a large mug.

Cucumber Mint Infused Water

YIELDS: 16 SERVINGS

Nutrients: 0.7 net carbs ~ 0.2g protein ~ 0g fats ~ 3 cal.

Ingredients:

1 med. cucumber

⅔ c. mint leaves

2 quarts water

How to prepare:

1. Toss the mint leaves into a pitcher. Press and mash the leaves gently.
2. Peel and slice the cucumber. Stir it into the water.
3. Let the pitcher rest in the fridge for a minimum of one hour.

Greek Iced Coffee

YIELDS: 1 SERVING

Nutrients: 10 net carbs ~ 3g protein ~ 1g fats ~ 57 cal.

Ingredients:

2 tsp. instant coffee

¼ c. cold water

1-2 tsp. sugar substitute

2 ice cubes

⅓ c. chilled milk

How to prepare:

1. Pour the water, ice cubes, sugar substitute, and coffee in a jar with a secure lid (a mason jar is perfect).
2. Shake vigorously until frothy, or for about 30 seconds. Add milk to the mix and enjoy!

Virgin Bloody Mary

YIELDS: 4 SERVINGS

Nutrients: 8 net carbs ~ 1g protein ~ 0g fats ~ 37 cal.

Ingredients:

3 large ripe tomatoes

2 jalapenos

¼ c. lemon juice

2-3 tsp. prepared horseradish

How to prepare:

1. Remove the stems and seeds from the jalapenos.
2. Slice the tomatoes into wedges and puree in a blender along with the horseradish, jalapenos, and lemon juice. Mix in the remainder of fixings and stir until well-blended.
3. Chill for two hours in the fridge.
4. Pour into chilled glasses along with ice and a spear of olives.

Smoothies

Blueberry Smoothie

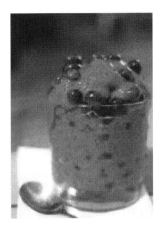

YIELDS: 1 SERVING

Nutrients: 3 net carbs ~ 31g protein ~ 21g fats ~ 343 cal.

Ingredients:

¼ c. blueberries

1 c. coconut milk

1 tbsp. vanilla essence

1 tbsp. MCT oil

Optional: 1 scoop whey protein powder

How to prepare:

1. Add the protein powder, blueberries, and the rest of the ingredients into the blender.
2. Toss in ice cubes and blend until creamy smooth.

Blueberry Yogurt Smoothie

YIELDS: 2 SERVINGS

Nutrients: 2 net carbs ~ 2g protein ~ 5g fats ~ 70 cal.

Ingredients:

10 blueberries

½ c. yogurt

½ tsp. vanilla extract

1 c. coconut milk

Stevia to taste

How to prepare:

1. Add all the fixings into the blender. Mix well.
2. When creamy, pour into two chilled mugs and enjoy.

Cinnamon Roll Smoothie

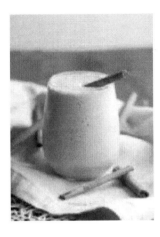

YIELDS: 1 SERVING

Nutrients: 0.6 net carbs ~ 26.5g protein ~ 3.25g fats ~ 145 cal.

Ingredients:

2 tbsp. vanilla protein powder

1 tsp. flax meal

1 c. almond milk

¼ tsp. vanilla extract

4 tsp. sweetener

½ tsp. cinnamon

1 c. ice

How to prepare:

1. Mix all the fixings in a blender. Empty the ice.

2. Blend using the high setting for 30 seconds or until thickened.

Mocha 5-Minute Smoothie

YIELDS: 3 SERVINGS

Nutrients: 4 net carbs ~ 3g protein ~ 16g fats ~ 176 cal.

Ingredients:

1½ c. unsweetened almond milk

½ c. coconut milk (from the can)

1 tsp. vanilla extract

2 tsp. instant coffee crystals (regular or decaffeinated)

3 tbsp. erythritol blend/granulated Stevia

3 tbsp. unsweetened cocoa powder

1 avocado

How to prepare:

1. Cut the avocado in half and remove the pit. Scoop out the center. Add it along with the rest of the ingredients into the blender.
2. Mix until smooth and serve.

Strawberry Avocado Smoothie

YIELDS: 2 SERVINGS

Nutrients: 11 net carbs ~ 2g protein ~ 14g fats ~ 165 cal.

Ingredients:

1 med. avocado

⅔ c. frozen strawberries

1 tbsp. lime juice

1½ c. coconut milk (in a carton for fewer carbs)

2 tsp. sugar equivalent OR ½ pkg. Stevia

½ c. ice (more or less)

How to prepare:

1. Mix the ingredients in a blender until creamy smooth.
2. Enjoy and serve in a couple of chilled glasses.

Other Tasty Selections

Avocado & Salmon Wrap

YIELDS: 2 SERVINGS

Nutrients: 5.8 net carbs ~ 36.9g protein ~ 66.9g fats ~ 765 cal.

Ingredients:

3 large eggs

½ pkg. smoked salmon (1.8 oz.)

½ average-sized avocado

1 spring onion

2 tbsp. cream cheese (full-fat)

2 tbsp. chives (freshly chopped)

1 tbsp. butter or ghee

To taste: pepper and salt

How to prepare:

1. In a mixing bowl, add a pinch of pepper and salt along with the eggs. Use a fork or whisk to mix well.
2. Chop and blend the chives and cream cheese.
3. Prepare the salmon and avocado (peel and slice).
4. In a skillet, add the butter or ghee along with the egg mixture. Cook until fluffy and soft.
5. Place the omelet on a serving dish and spoon the mixture of cheese over it.
6. Sprinkle the onion, prepared avocado, and salmon into the wrap. Close and enjoy!

Bacon Guacamole Fat Bombs

YIELDS: 6 SERVINGS

Nutrients: 1.4 net carbs ~ 3.4g protein ~ 15.2g fats ~ 156 cal.

Ingredients:

3½ oz. avocado (about ½ of large)

4 strips bacon

¼ c. butter or ghee

2 garlic cloves, crushed

½ small diced onion

1 small finely chopped chili pepper

1 tbsp. fresh lime juice (about ¼ of lime)

Salt as desired

Pinch ground black pepper or cayenne

1-2 tbsp. freshly chopped cilantro

How to prepare:

1. Program the oven setting to 375°F. Line the tray with parchment paper and cook the bacon for 10 to 15 minutes. Save the grease for step four.
2. Peel, deseed, and chop the avocado into a dish along with the garlic, chili pepper, lime juice, cilantro, black pepper, salt, and butter.
3. Use a fork or potato masher to combine the mixture and blend in the onion.

4. Empty the grease into the bomb, blend well, and cover for 20 to 30 minutes in the refrigerator. Make 6 balls.
5. Break up the bacon into a bowl and roll the balls in it until coated evenly. Serve for breakfast or a snack.

Bacon Baked Denver Omelet

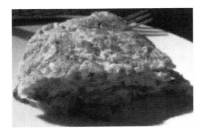

YIELDS: 4 SERVINGS

Nutrients: 3.6 net carbs ~ 22.4g protein ~ 26.8g fats ~345 cal.

Ingredients:

2 tbsp. butter

½ chopped green bell pepper

½ chopped onion

1 c. cooked chopped ham

¼ c. milk

8 eggs

½ c. shredded cheese

To taste: black pepper and salt

How to prepare:

1. Program the oven temperature to 400°F.
2. Lightly grease a 10-inch baking dish (round).
3. Over medium heat on the stovetop, use a large skillet to melt the butter. Toss in the onion and chopped pepper. Sauté for

approximately 5 minutes. Blend in the ham and cook another 5 minutes.

4. Beat the milk and eggs in a mixing container. Fold in the ham and cheese mixture. Shake in the pepper and salt. Empty into the casserole dish.

5. Bake about 25 minutes or until the eggs reach the desired consistency.

6. Serve and enjoy.

Banana Bread Muffins

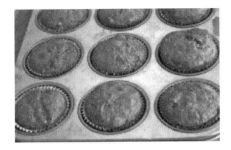

YIELDS: 12 SERVINGS

Nutrients: 11.2 net carbs ~ 4.9g protein ~ 11.6g fats ~ 165 cal.

Ingredients:

2½ c. mashed bananas (or 4-5 med.)

4 med. or 3 large eggs

¼ c. butter or olive oil

1 tsp. vanilla

½ c. almond or peanut butter

1 tbsp. cinnamon

1 pinch sea salt

½ c. coconut or almond flour

1 tsp. baking powder

1 tsp. baking soda

Optional: ½ c. chocolate chips (not included in nutritional facts)

Also needed: 12 muffin cups

How to prepare:

1. Set the oven temperature to 350°F. Use paper liners or grease the muffin tin.
2. Mix the bananas, eggs, butter, almond/peanut butter, and vanilla in a mixing dish. Whisk well and add the flour, baking soda, baking powder, a pinch of salt, and cinnamon. (It is best to stir using a wooden spoon until everything is well-mixed.)
3. Scoop the batter into the tins, approximately ¾ full.
4. Bake 15-18 minutes.
5. Cool for about 10 minutes before removing them from the tin.

Cheesy Omelet

YIELDS: 1 SERVING

Nutrients: 2.7 net carbs ~ 16.8g protein ~ 14.3g fats ~ 320 cal.

Ingredients:

1 tbsp. olive oil

2 large eggs

1 tbsp. milk (low-fat)

1/8 c. mozzarella cheese (low-fat, shredded)

¼ tsp. garlic powder

How to prepare:

1. Preheat a skillet on the medium-high setting. Add the oil.
2. Whisk the milk, eggs, and seasonings together. Pour the mixed ingredients into the hot pan. Swiftly prepare the eggs as if you were making scrambled eggs (avoid lumps).
3. As the mixture sets, cover the holes. When a light sheen appears over the top, spread the cheese over ½ the eggs.
4. Fold the opposite side over the cheesy side. Cook about 1 minute.
5. Serve.

Cream Cheese Pancakes

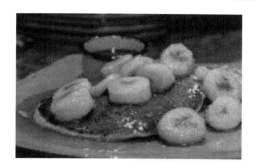

YIELDS: 7 SERVINGS

Nutrients: 0.9 net carbs ~ 7.2g protein ~ 12.7g fats ~ 149 cal.

Ingredients:

6 oz. cream cheese

4 duck eggs or 6 large hen eggs

Optional: 15 drops vanilla Stevia drops

1 tbsp. whole psyllium husks

How to prepare:

1. Combine all the fixings in a processor or small blender.
2. When creamy, add 3 tbsp. of the batter into a frying pan or hot griddle.
3. When it bubbles, flip and continue browning until done.
4. Garnish with your favorite low-carb toppings.

Egg Muffins

YIELDS: 6 MUFFINS

Nutrients: 1.1 net carbs ~ 11g protein ~ 13g fats ~ 148.6 cal.

Ingredients:

6 eggs

1 tbsp. olive oil

¼ c. diced onion

1 clove garlic

2 c. fresh spinach

¾ c. cheddar cheese (shredded, reduced-fat)

3 slices turkey bacon (chopped and cooked)

1 tbsp. milk

½ tsp. each:

Black pepper

Salt

How to prepare:

1. Place the oven setting at 350°F. Prepare a sauté pan using the oil.
2. Combine the onion and prepare using the medium heat setting for approximately 2 minutes. Blend the spinach with the onions until it wilts—roughly 2 or 3 more minutes.
3. Place the garlic in the pan and continue cooking for 30 seconds. Spice it with pepper and salt.

4. Whip the milk, cheese, and eggs in a separate dish. Toss in the bacon and spinach mixture.
5. Fill the muffin tins about ¾ full.
6. It's ready in 20 minutes or when the muffins are light brown around the edges.
7. Note: You can reheat them for 20 to 30 seconds in the microwave.

Guacamole Deviled Eggs

YIELDS: 8 SERVINGS

Nutrients: 5 net carbs ~ 4.2g protein ~ 9.9g fats ~ 119 cal.

Ingredients:

4 eggs (in the shell)

1 tbsp. minced green onion

1 tbsp. chopped cilantro

2 avocados (peeled, pitted, and mashed)

2 tsp. fresh lime juice

2 tsp. seeded jalapeno pepper

1 dash hot pepper sauce (Tabasco)

½ tsp. salt

1 tsp. Worcestershire sauce

1 tsp. Dijon-style mustard

Pinch paprika

How to prepare:

1. Gently place the eggs in a saucepan. Submerge in fresh water. Place a lid on the pot and let it simmer for 10-12 minutes.
2. Transfer the eggs from the pot and let them cool in a container of cold water. When chilled, slice into halves and add the yolks to a mixing container. Toss in the cilantro, avocado, jalapeno, and onion.
3. Stir in the juice along with the mustard, Worcestershire sauce, salt,

and hot sauce. Blend well.

4. Fill the egg white halves and stick in the fridge until ready to eat.
5. Sprinkle with the paprika.

Hot Dish: Sausage, Egg, & Cheese

YIELDS: 12 SERVINGS

Nutrients: 4.1 net carbs ~ 13.6g protein ~ 34.3g fats ~ 151 cal.

Ingredients:

½ lb. ground pork

10 med. eggs

6 slices bread

1½ c. milk

1/8 tsp. mustard

4 oz. cheddar cheese (shredded)

½ tsp. each:

Salt

Pepper

Also needed: 9x13 casserole dish

How to prepare:

1. Cook the sausage and drain. Toast the bread on a lightly greased baking dish.
2. Scramble the eggs and mix with the milk. Add the mustard, salt, and pepper as you like. Fold in the crumbled sausage and mix.
3. Pour the mixture over the toast. Add the cheese and let it set in the fridge overnight.
4. The next morning, warm up the oven to 350°F. Let the dish reach

room temperature.

5. Bake the prepared dish for 25 minutes or until done.

Individual Baked Eggs

———

YIELDS: 1 SERVING

Nutrients: 0.6 net carbs ~ 10.7g protein ~ 14.3g fats ~ 174 cal.

Ingredients:

1 tsp. melted butter

1 slice bacon

1 egg

¼ slice cheese

How to prepare:

1. Set the oven temperature to 350°F.
2. Cook the bacon using the medium-high heat setting on the stovetop. It should be browned but flexible.
3. Wrap a muffin cup with the prepared bacon. Drop in the butter, then the egg.
4. Bake for 10-15 minutes. Enjoy.

Mexican Breakfast Casserole (Crockpot)

YIELDS: 10 SERVINGS

Nutrients: 5.2 net carbs ~ 17.9g protein ~ 24.1g fats ~ 320 cal.

Ingredients:

1 pkg. (12 oz.) pork sausage roll

1 tsp. each:

Chili powder

Cumin

½ tsp. each:

Coriander

Garlic powder

¼ tsp. each:

Pepper

Salt

1 c. salsa

10 eggs

1 c. each:

Pepper Jack or your choice of cheese

1% milk

Optional Toppings:

Cilantro

Salsa

Sour cream

Avocado

How to prepare:

1. On the stovetop, use a skillet over medium heat to cook the sausage. Add the salsa and seasonings. When done, set aside to slightly cool.
2. Whisk the milk and eggs in another dish. Add the mixtures together and toss in the cheese. Mix well.
3. Coat the bottom of the cooker with a little cooking spray and empty in the fixings.
4. Secure the lid and cook using the high setting for 2.5 hours or on low for 5 hours.
5. Add the desired toppings.

Mini Ham Rolls

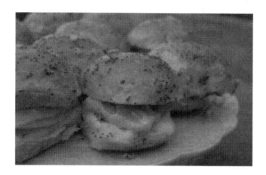

YIELDS: 24 SERVINGS

Nutrients: 10.2 net carbs ~ 5.7g protein ~ 9g fats ~ 145 cal.

Ingredients:

2 tbsp. each:

Dried minced onions

Poppy seeds

1 tbsp. prepared mustard

½ c. melted margarine

24 dinner rolls

½ lb. each:

Thinly sliced Swiss cheese

Chopped ham

How to prepare:

1. Set the oven temperature in advance to 325°F.

2. Mix the mustard, onion flakes, margarine, and poppy seeds in a small mixing dish.
3. Make sandwiches with the ham, cheese, and dinner rolls. Place them on a baking sheet. Drizzle the poppy seed mix over the top.
4. Bake until the cheese has melted (20 minutes or so).

Pumpkin Maple Flaxseed Muffins

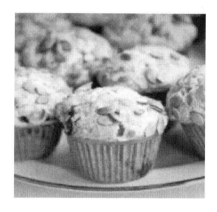

YIELDS: 10 SERVINGS

Nutrients: 2 net carbs ~ 5g protein ~ 8.5g fats ~ 120 cal.

Ingredients:

1¼ c. ground flaxseeds

½ tbsp. baking powder

⅓ c. erythritol

1 tbsp. each:

Cinnamon

Pumpkin pie spice

½ tsp. salt

2 tbsp. coconut oil

1 c. pure pumpkin puree

1 egg

½ tsp. each:

Vanilla extract

Apple cider vinegar

¼ c. maple syrup

Topping: Pumpkin seeds

Useful appliances: Blender such as NutriBullet

How to prepare:

1. Set the oven temperature to 350°F. Prepare a muffin tin (10 sections) with silicone cupcake liners.
2. Add the seeds to the NutriBullet for about 1 second—any longer and it could become damp.
3. Combine the dry fixings and whisk until well-mixed. Add the puree, vanilla extract, and pumpkin spice. Add the maple syrup (½ tsp.) if using.
4. Blend in the oil, egg, and vinegar. Combine nuts or any other fold-ins of your choice but add the carbs or calories.
5. Scoop out the mixture by the tablespoon into the prepared tins. Garnish with some of the pumpkin seeds. Leave a little space at the top because they will rise.
6. Bake approximately 20 minutes. They are ready when they are slightly browned. Let them cool a few minutes. Add some ghee/butter.

Quiche Cups

YIELDS: 1-2 SERVINGS

Nutrients: 2.1 net carbs ~ 12.8g protein ~ 14.2g fats ~ 105 cal.

2 c. frozen spinach

½ an onion

2 c. Egg Beaters

½ c. mozzarella cheese, shredded

½ tsp. hot sauce

How to prepare:

1. Prepare a muffin tin with cooking spray or a paper liner.
2. Chop the spinach and slice the onion. Microwave both until the onion is soft and the spinach is thawed.
3. Combine everything and sprinkle with the pepper and salt.
4. Bake at 375°F for 20 minutes.

Chapter 8: Lunchtime Specialties

Bacon & Shrimp Risotto

YIELDS: 2 SERVINGS

Nutrients: 5.3 net carbs ~23.7g protein ~ 9.4g fats ~224 cal.

Ingredients:

4 slices chopped bacon

2 c. daikon/winter radish

2 tbsp. dry white wine

¼ c. chicken stock

1 minced garlic clove

To taste: Ground pepper

2 tbsp. chopped parsley

4 oz. cooked shrimp

How to prepare:

1. Peel and slice the daikon/radish, mince the garlic, and chop the bacon. Remove as much water as possible from the daikon once it's shredded.
2. On the stovetop, warm up a saucepan using the medium heat setting. Toss in the bacon and fry until crispy. Leave the drippings in the pan and remove the bacon with a slotted spoon to drain.
3. Add the wine, daikon, salt, pepper, stock, and garlic into the pan. Cook 6-8 minutes until most of the liquid is absorbed.
4. Fold in the bacon (save a few bits for the topping) and shrimp along with the parsley.
5. Serve and enjoy.

6. Note: If you cannot find daikon, substitute some shredded cauliflower in its place.

Baked Zucchini Noodles with Feta

YIELDS: 3 SERVINGS

Nutrients: 5 net carbs ~ 4g protein ~ 8g fats ~ 105 cal.

Ingredients:

1 plum tomato

2 zucchinis

8 cubes feta cheese

1 tsp. each:

Pepper

Salt

1 tbsp. olive oil

How to prepare:

1. Grease a roasting pan. Program the oven to 375°F.
2. Slice the tomato into quarters. Prepare the noodles with a spiralizer and add to the prepared pan along with the olive oil and tomatoes. Sprinkle with the pepper and salt.
3. Bake for 10-15 minutes. Transfer from the oven and add the cheese cubes, tossing to combine. Serve.

BBQ Pork for Sandwiches (Slow Cooker)

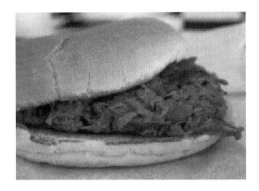

YIELDS: 12 SERVINGS

Nutrients: 5.1 net carbs ~ 30.3g protein ~ 18.1g fats ~ 313 cal.

Ingredients:

3 lb. pork ribs, boneless

1 can (14 oz.) beef broth

1 c. shredded carrot (canned is okay)

4½ oz. each sauce:

Mesquite

Barbecue

How to prepare:

1. Empty the ribs and beef broth into the slow cooker.
2. Set the pot on high for approximately 4 hours or until the meat is easily shredded.
3. Remove when done and use two forks to shred the pork.
4. Serve any time for a tasty sandwich.

Beef Stew

YIELDS: 6 SERVINGS

Nutrients: 9 net carbs ~ 27g protein ~ 10g fats ~ 222 cal.

Ingredients:

1 pkg. (5 lbs.) stew beef

2 cans chili-ready diced tomatoes (14.5 oz. each)

1 c. beef broth

1 tbsp. each:

Chili mix (pre-packaged)

Worcestershire sauce

2 tsp. hot sauce

Salt to taste

How to prepare:

1. Use the high setting on the slow cooker and toss in all the fixings.
2. Prepare for 6 hours. Break apart the meat and cook for an additional 2 hours. Add a pinch of salt.
3. Serve and enjoy your lunch!

Broccoli & Tuna

YIELDS: 2 SERVINGS

Nutrients: 3 net carbs ~ 14.2g protein ~ 20.6g fats ~ 122 cal.

Ingredients:

1 3-oz. can light tuna

1 c. broccoli

2 tbsp. cheese

1 tsp. salt

How to prepare:

1. Place the frozen florets of broccoli in water until they are thawed. Drain.
2. Mix the broccoli and the cheese until melted. Fold in the tuna.
3. Salt if desired.
4. Serve any time for a great treat.

Caprese Salad

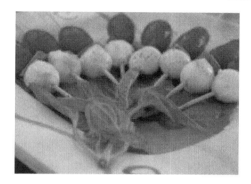

YIELDS: 4 SERVINGS

Nutrients: 4.58 net carbs ~ 7.7g protein ~ 63g fats ~ 191 cal.

Ingredients:

3 c. grape tomatoes

4 peeled garlic cloves

2 tbsp. avocado oil

10 pearl-sized mozzarella balls

4 c. baby spinach leaves

¼ c. fresh basil leaves

1 tbsp. each:

Brine (reserved from the cheese)

Pesto

How to prepare:

1. Use aluminum foil to cover a baking tray.
2. Program the oven to 400°F.
3. Arrange the cloves and tomatoes on the baking pan and drizzle with the oil. Bake 20-30 minutes until the tops are slightly browned.
4. Drain the liquid (saving 1 tbsp.) from the mozzarella. Mix the pesto with the brine.
5. Arrange the spinach in a large serving bowl. Transfer the tomatoes to the dish along with the roasted garlic. Drizzle with the pesto sauce.
6. Garnish with the mozzarella balls and freshly torn basil leaves.
7. A great treat for lunch! Add them to skewers for a change.

Cauliflower & Shrimp Salad

YIELD: 6 1 C. SERVINGS

Nutrients: 5 net carbs ~ 17g protein ~ 13g fats ~ 214 cal.

Ingredients:

1 lb. med. raw shrimp

1 head cauliflower

2 cucumbers

1 tbsp. & ¼ c. olive oil

3 tbsp. freshly chopped dill

2 tbsp. grated lemon zest

¼ c. fresh lemon juice

How to prepare:

1. Peel, clean, and discard the tail from the shrimp. Arrange them on a baking tin and sprinkle with 1 tbsp. of the oil.
2. Roast at 350°F for approximately 8-10 minutes. Remove when opaque.
3. Chop the cauliflower into small pieces and discard the head.
4. Microwave the florets in a shallow bowl for 5 minutes until they have a soft texture—not mushy. Let cool.
5. Peel, remove the seed, and chop the cucumbers into ½-inch pieces.
6. After the shrimp have cooled, slice them lengthwise or chop them up.
7. Combine the cucumber, cauliflower, and the shrimp. Add the chopped dill and lemon zest.
8. Note: Hold the ¼ c. lemon juice or the remainder of the olive oil (¼

c.) mixture that will be used as the dressing.

Chicken Korma (Instant Pot)

YIELDS: 6 SERVINGS

Nutrients: 6 net carbs ~ 14g protein ~ 19g fats ~ 256 cal.

Ingredients:

1 lb. chicken thighs

½ c. diced tomatoes

1 chopped onion

½ jalapeno/green serrano

5 garlic cloves

1 tsp. each:

Garam masala

Salt

Turmeric

Minced ginger

½ tsp. each:

Ground coriander

Cayenne pepper

Ground cumin

½ c. water

Ingredients for the finish:

½ c. unsweetened coconut milk

1 tsp. garam masala

¼ c. chopped cilantro

How to prepare:

1. Combine all the veggies and spices. Add to the Instant Pot.
2. Toss in the chicken and set the timer for 10 minutes (high-pressure). Naturally release the steam.
3. Remove the chicken and dice. Pour in the garam masala and coconut milk along with the chicken in the pot. Warm it for a couple of minutes.
4. Garnish and serve.

Chicken Stir Fry

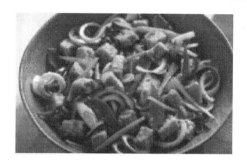

YIELDS: 4 SERVINGS

Nutrients: 4 net carbs ~ 27g protein ~ 10g fats ~ 220 cal.

Ingredients:

1 whole zucchini

4 chicken breasts

½ c. grape tomatoes

1 yellow onion

1 tsp. each:

Black pepper

Salt

2 tbsp. coconut oil

How to prepare:

1. Do the prep: Slice the chicken into cubes. Slice or julienne the zucchini. Chop the onion and cut the tomatoes into halves.
2. Warm up a skillet using medium heat and add the coconut oil.

3. Place the chicken in the pan and sauté until done (7-10 minutes).
4. Toss in the rest of the fixings and continue cooking until the zucchini is tender. Add other garnishes to your liking, but add the carbs. Serve.

Fresh Lobster Salad

———

YIELDS: 4 SERVINGS

Nutrients: 1.1 net carbs ~ 21.6g protein ~ 23.4g fats ~303 cal.

Ingredients:

¼ c. each:

Melted butter

Mayonnaise

1 lb. cooked lobster meat

⅛ tsp. black pepper

How to prepare:

1. Chop the lobster into bite-sized pieces. Melt and pour the butter over the meat.
2. Toss to coat and blend in the mayonnaise along with the pepper.
3. Chill in a covered dish for a minimum of 20 minutes.

Greek Tuna Salad

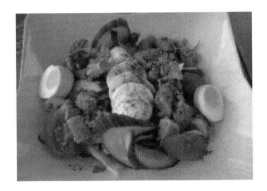

YIELDS: 6 SERVINGS

Nutrients: 7 net carbs ~ 20g protein ~ 16g fats ~ 169 cal.

Ingredients:

1 18-oz. can chunk light tuna (packed in water)

6 oz. pepperoncini

9 c. romaine lettuce

2 c. cucumber

1 c. cherry tomatoes

¾ c. each:

Feta cheese crumbles (reduced-fat)

Red onion

18 sliced black olives

Optional: 1 boiled egg

Ingredients for the Zesty Dressing (optional):

1½ tsp. oregano

¼ c. olive oil

½ tsp. black pepper

2 tbsp. red wine vinegar

Optional: ½ tsp. salt

How to prepare:

1. Do the prep: Drain and slice the pepperoncini. Peel and dice the cucumber. Chop the tomatoes into halves and slice the onion into rings.
2. Mix all ingredients for the salad (first list).
3. Combine all the fixings for the dressing (optional). Enjoy with an added boiled egg.
4. Note: The dressing and egg are not calculated in nutrition counts.

Hot & Sour Soup (Instant Pot)

YIELDS: 8 SERVINGS

Nutrients: 5 net carbs ~ 20g protein ~ 5g fats ~ 158 cal.

Ingredients:

1 lb. thinly sliced pork tenderloin

5 c. low-sodium chicken broth

1 tbsp. Chinese black or white vinegar

2 tbsp. Chinese rice or white vinegar

3 tbsp. soy sauce or coconut aminos

1 c. dried "wood-ear" mushrooms

½ tsp. xanthan gum

2 tsp. pepper

1 tsp. salt

3 tbsp. water

Ingredients after the soup is cooked:

4 lightly beaten eggs

1 lb. extra-firm tofu

How to prepare:

1. Add all the fixings into the Instant Pot (omit eggs and tofu for now).
2. Use the soup function for 10 minutes (high pressure). Naturally release the pressure for 15 minutes, then use quick release. Keep it

warm using the sauté function.

3. Remove the mushrooms and slice thinly. Add them back to the pot. Dice the tofu and add the eggs.

4. Stir with chopsticks and let it sauté for a minute before serving.

Mexican Chicken Avocado Salad

YIELDS: 4 SERVINGS

Nutrients: 9.8 net carbs ~ 23.5g protein ~ 16.3g fats ~ 277 cal.

Ingredients:

2 chicken breasts, boneless

1 jalapeno

1 red bell pepper

⅓ red onion

⅛ c. cilantro

1 diced avocado

1 tbsp. lime juice

¼ c. plain Greek yogurt

2 tbsp. ranch dressing

1 tsp. pepper

1½ tsp. garlic powder

½ tsp. each:

Salt

Chili powder

How to prepare:

1. Heat a pot of water with ½ teaspoon of salt to boiling. Simmer the

chicken for approximately 40 minutes if frozen and 20 minutes if the chicken is fresh.

2. Slice or dice up the veggies and finely chop the cilantro in a mixing dish.
3. In another container, combine the ranch, yogurt, spices, lime juice, and avocado.
4. Dice or shred the chicken when done.
5. Combine all the fixings. Chill for a minimum of 4 hours so all the ingredients can mix well.
6. Serve on a platter of lettuce or as a sandwich wrap.

Parmesan Broccoli Balls

YIELDS: 36 SERVINGS

Nutrients: 4.2 net carbs ~ 2.4g protein ~ 5.1g fats ~ 71 cal.

Ingredients:

1 pkg. frozen broccoli (10 oz.)

1 pkg. stuffing mix chicken flavor (6 oz.)

1 med. chopped onion

1 tsp. ground black pepper

½ tsp. garlic salt

½ c. grated parmesan cheese

¾ c. melted margarine

6 eggs, whisked

How to prepare:

1. Thaw the broccoli. Prepare a saucepan with enough water to cover the broccoli. Let it boil with a lid for 5 minutes. Remove the top and simmer another 2-3 minutes. Drain well and let it cool.
2. Combine the broccoli with the remainder of the fixings in a large mixing bowl. Place the top on the container and chill for at least an hour. The moisture should be absorbed.
3. Warm up the oven to 325°F.
4. Roll the mixture into 1-inch balls and place on a baking sheet.
5. Bake until browned or for 15-20 minutes.

Pork Vegetables & Noodles (Instant Pot)

YIELDS: 6 SERVINGS

Nutrients: 3 net carbs ~15g protein ~ 18g fats ~ 241 cal.

Ingredients:

1 tbsp. oil

1 lb. ground pork

1 c. chopped bell peppers

2 garlic cloves

½ c. chopped onion

4 c. chopped baby spinach

2 pkg. shirataki noodles

½ c. grated parmesan cheese

How to prepare:

1. Warm up the Instant Pot using the sauté function. Add the oil when hot.
2. Toss in the pork and sauté until slightly pink. Add the garlic, onions, peppers, and spinach. Scrape the browning bits from the bottom and secure the lid.
3. Use the high-pressure setting for 3 minutes and quick release the pressure.
4. Empty the sauce over the noodles and garnish with cheese.

Roasted Celery & Macadamia Cheese

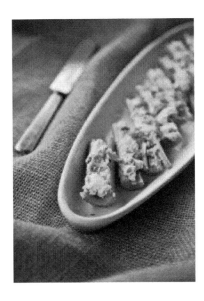

YIELDS: 5 SERVINGS

Nutrients: 2.38 net carbs ~ 2.43g protein ~ 13g fats ~ 139.6 cal.

Ingredients:

3 tbsp. nutritional yeast

6 oz. macadamia nuts

5 large celery stalks

½ c. water

2 tbsp. lemon juice

To taste: Pepper and salt

½ tsp. garlic powder

5 leaves fresh basil

How to prepare:

1. Program the oven to 350°F.
2. Rinse the celery and cut into halves. Remove the strings.
3. Process the lemon juice, nuts, yeast, water, garlic powder, and basil. Shake in the pepper and salt.
4. Spoon the cheese into the stalks (removing as many strings as you can).
5. Bake 40 minutes. For a charred look, place under the broiler for a minute or so.
6. When it's ready, slice it with a fork.

Spinach Quiche

YIELDS: 8 SERVINGS

Nutrients: 6.1 net carbs ~ 19.1g protein ~ 14.9g fats ~ 231 cal.

Ingredients:

1 pkg. (10 oz.) of frozen and thawed spinach

1 bunch green onions

1 container (16 oz.) cottage cheese

4 beaten eggs

2 c. shredded cheddar cheese

¼ c. crushed croutons

Also needed: 1 9-inch pie or quiche pan

How to prepare:

1. Finely chop the onions (white segments only) and the spinach.
2. Warm up the oven to 325°F. Lightly grease the chosen pan.
3. Use a small pan over the medium stovetop setting. Cook the spinach until softened. Drain the liquid. Add the eggs and onions along with the cottage and cheddar cheeses.
4. Empty the mixture into the pan. Bake for 45 minutes. Remove and sprinkle with the croutons. Bake another 15 minutes or until your eggs are cooked as desired.

Spinach Salad

YIELDS: 1 SERVING

Nutrients: 3.5 net carbs ~ 8g protein ~18g fats ~ 208 cal.

Ingredients:

3 c. spinach

2 tbsp. ranch dressing

½ tsp. diced red pepper

1½ tbsp. parmesan cheese

How to prepare:

1. Arrange the spinach in a salad container.
2. Drizzle with the dressing, red pepper, and cheese.
3. Toss well and enjoy.

Stuffed Mushrooms

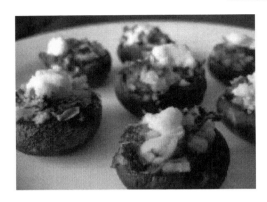

YIELDS: 12 SERVINGS

Nutrients: 1.5 net carbs ~ 2.7g protein ~ 8.2g fats ~ 88 cal.

Ingredients:

12 fresh whole mushrooms

1 tbsp. each:

Minced garlic

Vegetable oil

¼ c. grated parmesan cheese

1 pkg. (8 oz.) softened cream cheese

¼ tsp. each:

Onion powder

Ground cayenne pepper

Ground black pepper

How to prepare:

1. Program the oven to 350°F.
2. Clean the mushrooms with a damp paper towel and break off the stems, trimming away any rough ends.
3. Prepare a baking sheet with cooking spray.
4. Warm up the oil using the medium heat option. Toss the chopped mushroom stems and garlic into the skillet with the oil. Cook until the moisture is absorbed. Set aside to cool.
5. Blend the mixture with the cream cheese, cayenne pepper, parmesan cheese, onion powder, and black pepper. Fill each of the mushroom caps. Arrange on the baking tin.
6. Bake for 20 minutes until the mushrooms are steaming hot.

Chapter 9: Dinnertime Meals

Asian-Style Tuna Patties

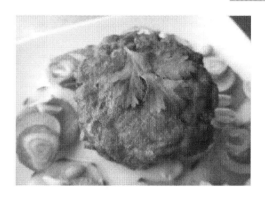

YIELDS: 6 PATTIES

Nutrients: 3.8 net carbs ~ 17.7g protein ~ 4.2g fats ~ 145 cal.

Ingredients:

2 cans light tuna

1 tsp. sesame oil

2 slices bread, wheat reduced-calorie OR ¾ c. dried breadcrumbs

¼ c. egg substitute (Egg Beaters is excellent)

1 clove garlic

3 green onions

1 tsp. black pepper

Non-stick cooking spray

1 tbsp. each of:

Teriyaki sauce

Ketchup

Soy sauce

How to prepare:

1. For the breadcrumbs: Bake the slices of bread at 200°F until dried out. Put in a blender or food processor to equal ¾ cup.
2. Do the prep: Drain the tuna. Peel and mince the garlic and onions. Mix the egg, tuna, breadcrumbs, garlic, and green onions in a large bowl.
3. Blend the teriyaki sauce, soy sauce, ketchup, pepper, and sesame oil into the mixture.
4. Shape the tuna patties into 1-inch thickness.
5. Over medium heat in a greased pan with a bit of non-stick cooking spray, fry each side for approximately 5 minutes.
6. Enjoy with your favorite side dish.

Baked Tilapia with Cherry Tomatoes

YIELDS: 2 SERVINGS

Nutrients: 4 net carbs ~ 23g protein ~ 8g fats ~ 180 cal.

Ingredients:

2 tsp. butter

2 (4 oz.) tilapia fillets

8 cherry tomatoes

¼ c. pitted black olives

1 tsp. garlic powder

¼ tsp. each:

Black pepper

Paprika

½ tsp. salt

1 tbsp. lemon juice, freshly squeezed

Optional: 1 tbsp. balsamic vinegar

How to prepare:

1. Set the oven to 375°F.
2. Grease a roasting pan and add the butter along with the olives and tomatoes on the bottom.
3. Season the tilapia with the spices (paprika, salt, pepper, and garlic powder). Add the fish fillets with the lemon juice.
4. Cover the pan with foil and bake until the fish easily flakes (25-30

minutes).

5. Garnish with the vinegar if desired.

Balsamic Chicken Thighs

YIELDS: 8 SERVINGS

Nutrients: 3.6 net carbs ~ 20.1g protein ~ 4g fats ~ 133 cal.

Ingredients:

8 boneless chicken thighs (approx 24 oz..)

4 minced cloves garlic

2 tsp. dried minced onion

1 tbsp. extra-virgin olive oil

1 tsp. each:

Garlic powder

Dried basil

½ tsp. each:

Pepper

Salt

½ c. balsamic vinegar

Sprinkle of freshly chopped parsley

How to prepare:

1. Mix all the dry spices (minced onion, pepper, salt, basil, and garlic powder). Rub over the chicken and set aside.
2. Pour the extra-virgin olive oil and garlic into the slow cooker. Add the chicken.

3. Empty the vinegar over the thighs. Securely close the lid.
4. Cook for 4 hours using the high-temperature setting.
5. Sprinkle with the freshly chopped parsley, serve, and enjoy.

Barbacoa Beef

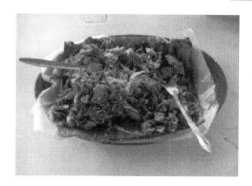

YIELDS: 9 SERVINGS

Nutrients: 2 net carbs ~ 24g protein ~ 4.5g fats ~ 153 cal.

Ingredients:

½ med. onion

5 garlic cloves

2-4 chipotles in adobo sauce (to taste)

1 lime, juiced

1 tbsp. each (ground):

Cumin

Oregano

1 c. water

½ tsp. ground cloves

3 bay leaves

2½ tsp. kosher salt

Black pepper (to taste)

3 lb. eye of round/bottom round

1 tsp. oil

How to prepare:

1. In a blender, puree the onion, garlic cloves, lime juice, water, cloves, chipotles, cumin, and oregano until smooth.
2. Remove all fat from the meat and chop into 3-inch bits. Season with 2 tsp. of salt and a pinch of pepper.
3. Prepare the Instant Pot on the sauté setting and add the oil. Brown the meat in batches (5 minutes). Into the Instant Pot, add the sauce from the blender along with the bay leaves.
4. Secure the lid and set the timer for 65 minutes using the high-pressure setting. Natural or quick release the pressure and shred the beef with two forks. Reserve the juices and throw the bay leaves in the bin.
5. Return the meat to the pot with the cumin, salt to taste, and 1½ cups of the reserved juices. Serve while hot.

Braised Cube Steak

———

YIELDS: 8 SERVINGS

Nutrients: 3 net carbs ~ 23.5g protein ~ 5.5g fats ~ 154 cal.

Ingredients:

1 c. water

8 cubed steaks (28-oz. pkg.)

Black pepper to taste

1¾ tsp. garlic salt or adobo seasoning

1 can tomato sauce (8 oz.)

⅓ c. green pitted olives + 2 tbsp. brine

1 small red pepper

½ med. onion

How to prepare:

1. Chop the peppers and onions into ¼-inch strips.
2. Prepare the beef with the salt/adobo and pepper. Toss into the Instant Pot with the remainder of the fixings.
3. Secure the top and prepare for 25 minutes under high pressure. Natural release the pressure and serve.

Chicken Teriyaki

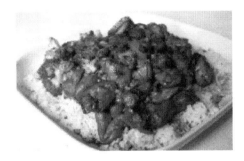

YIELDS: 6 SERVINGS

Nutrients: 4 net carbs ~ 20g protein ~ 6g fats ~ 158 cal.

Ingredients:

2 lb. chicken thighs

2 red peppers (spicy)

1 yellow onion

3 garlic cloves

½ c. reduced-sodium beef broth

¼ c. coconut aminos

⅓ c. water

1 1-inch knob of freshly grated ginger

To taste: Pepper and salt

For the garnish: 4 green onions

Optional for serving: Lettuce leaves

How to prepare:

1. Prep the veggies: Chop the peppers, onions, and garlic.
2. Whisk the water, aminos, and broth. Add to the cooker. Blend in the rest of the fixings (omitting the lettuce and green onions).
3. Cook for 6 hours using the high-heat setting.
4. When done, garnish with the green onion as-is OR on a bed of lettuce to create a tasty taco. Enjoy with a side of broccoli.

Grilled Buffalo Chicken Lettuce Wraps

YIELDS: 15-20 BUTTERCUP servings

Nutrients: 2 net carbs ~ 5g protein ~ 3g fats ~ 53 cal.

Ingredients:

¾ c. Frank's RedHot Sauce

3 large boneless & skinless breasts of chicken

15-20 lettuce cups

1 diced avocado

¾ c. cherry tomatoes

½ c. ranch dressing

¼ c. sliced green onions

Also needed: Grill basket or kabob sticks

How to prepare:

1. Dice up the chicken into ½-inch cubes. Slice the tomatoes into halves. Set aside.
2. Place the chicken in a dish and add Frank's RedHot Sauce (or your choice of hot sauce). Put a lid or foil over the container. Put it in the refrigerator for about 30 minutes.
3. Set the grill temperature to 400°F.
4. Arrange the grill basket with the chicken/kabobs on the grill and cook for 8-10 minutes. Stir constantly. Remove them from the grill and dump into a container with the remainder of the buffalo sauce.
5. Prepare the lettuce cups with 2 or 3 cubes of chicken, 2 or 3 diced tomatoes, a pinch of onions, 2 or 3 diced avocados, and a drizzle of

dressing.

6. Enjoy your healthy masterpiece!

Grilled Chicken with Spinach & Mozzarella

YIELDS: 6 SERVINGS

Nutrients: 3.7 net carbs ~ 30.9g protein ~ 6.1g fats ~ 195 cal.

Ingredients:

3 large chicken breasts (24 oz.) or 6 portions

1 tsp. olive oil

Pepper and kosher salt to taste

3 crushed garlic cloves

10 oz. drained frozen spinach

½ c. roasted red pepper (strips packed in water)

3 oz. shredded part-skim mozzarella

Olive oil cooking spray

How to prepare:

1. Warm the oven to 400°F. Prepare the grill/grill pan with the oil.
2. Sprinkle the salt and pepper onto the chicken. Cook about 2-3 minutes per side.
3. Add the oil into a frying pan along with the garlic. Continue cooking for about 30 seconds. Add a sprinkle of salt and pepper. Toss in the spinach. Sauté another 2-3 minutes.
4. Arrange the chicken on a baking sheet and add the spinach to each. Top them off with 1/2 the cheese and peppers. Bake about 3 minutes until lightly toasted.
5. Serve a slice of delight!

Ground Beef Eggplant Casserole (Slow Cooker)

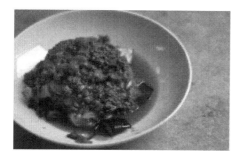

YIELDS: 12 SERVINGS

Nutrients: 5.7 net carbs ~ 15.9g protein ~ 12.8g fats ~209 cal.

Ingredients:

2 lb. ground beef

2 c. cubed eggplant

1 tbsp. olive oil

2 tsp. salt

½ tsp. pepper

2 tsp. each:

Mustard

Worcestershire sauce

1 can each:

28 oz. drained diced tomatoes

16 oz. canned tomato sauce

2 c. grated mozzarella cheese

1 tsp. oregano

2 tbsp. parsley

How to prepare:

1. Sprinkle the salt over the sliced eggplant and let it rest for 30 minutes or so. Add to a bowl and coat with oil.
2. Combine the beef, pepper, salt, mustard, and Worcestershire sauce. Mash into the base of the pan and top with the eggplant. Spread out the tomatoes and sauce. Drizzle with the rest of the fixings.
3. Prepare on the high setting for 2-3 hours or on low for 3-4 hours.

Herbal Green Beans & Chicken

YIELDS: 3 SERVINGS

Nutrients: 4 net carbs ~ 19g protein ~ 11g fats ~ 196 cal.

Ingredients:

2 tbsp. olive oil

1 c. trimmed green beans

2 whole chicken breasts

8 halved cherry tomatoes

1 tbsp. Italian seasoning

1 tsp. each:

Salt

Pepper

How to prepare:

1. Warm up a skillet using the medium heat setting. Add the oil.
2. Sprinkle the chicken with the pepper, Italian seasoning, and salt.
3. Arrange in the skillet for 10 minutes per side, or until thoroughly done. Add the tomatoes and beans. Simmer another 5-7 minutes and serve.

Korean Spicy Pork

YIELDS: 4 SERVINGS

Nutrients: 9 net carbs ~ 15g protein ~ 9g fats ~ 189 cal.

Ingredients:

1 lb. pork shoulder

1 thinly sliced onion

1 tbsp. each:

Minced garlic

Minced ginger

Soy sauce

Sesame oil

Rice wine

2 Splenda packs

1 tsp. cayenne

2 tbsp. gochugaru

¼ c. water

Ingredients for finishing:

¼ c. sliced green onion

1 tbsp. sesame seeds

1 thinly sliced onion

How to prepare:

1. Cut the pork into ¼- to ½-inch slices. Add the rest of the marinade ingredients into a container. Let this rest for 1 to 24 hours. When ready to cook, use the high-pressure setting for 20 minutes. Naturally release.
2. Use a cast-iron skillet to cook the thinly sliced onion and pork cubes. Once the pan is hot, empty in the sauce and mix with the pork.
3. When the sauce has cooled down, the onions will be soft. Toss the green onions and sesame seeds. Serve.

Miso Salmon

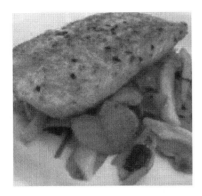

YIELDS: 4 SERVINGS

Nutrients: 0.78 net carbs ~ 28.38g protein ~ 9.23g fats ~ 215 cal.

Ingredients:

1 ¼-lb. salmon fillets (skin on)

2 tbsp. white wine

3 tbsp. each:

Sake

Miso (white suggested)

To taste: Kosher salt

How to prepare:

1. Slice the salmon into fillets and sprinkle with the salt. Rest for 30 minutes to help remove some of the moisture. Gently wipe off the salt with a towel with 1 tbsp. of the sake.
2. Mix the white wine, miso, and rest of the sake into a dish.

3. Pour approximately ⅓ of the marinade into an airtight bowl. Add the fillets and the rest of the marinade. Refrigerate for 1 to 2 days.
4. When ready to eat, warm up the oven to 400°F. Cover a baking tin with parchment paper.
5. Scrape away the marinade with your fingers to help prevent burning.
6. Bake for 25 minutes and serve.

Pan-Glazed Chicken & Basil

YIELDS: 4 SERVINGS

Nutrients: 4.6 net carbs ~ 26.2g protein ~ 4.7g fats ~ 161 cal.

Ingredients:

4 chicken breast halves (4 oz.)

2 tbsp. balsamic vinegar

2 tsp. each:

Olive oil

Dried basil

¼ tsp. each:

Salt

Black pepper

1 tbsp. honey

How to prepare:

1. Spice up the chicken with sea salt or a coarser salt. You can also add pepper.
2. Place the chicken in a large pan with oil on a medium-high burner. Usually, 4 or 5 minutes on each side is sufficient.
3. Flip the chicken and simmer for an extra 5 minutes or so.
4. Blend in the vinegar, basil, and honey; continue cooking for 1 minute.

Pork & Green Pepper Kabobs

YIELDS: 4 SERVINGS

Nutrients: 5 net carbs ~ 24g protein ~ 8g fats ~ 200 cal.

Ingredients:

2 tbsp. hot sauce

3 tbsp. butter

½ tsp. crushed red pepper

1 tbsp. each:

Minced garlic

Soy sauce

Water

1 lb. pork kabob squares

1 med. green pepper

How to prepare:

1. Combine all the marinade fixings in a food processor. Run until creamy smooth. Cut the pork into bite-sized squares and place them in a plastic or ceramic container. Mix the marinade with the chicken and let it rest from 1 to 24 hours.
2. Chop the peppers into small bits along with the pork. Thread them onto metal skewers. Broil for 5 minutes on each side until the internal temperature reaches 145°F.
3. Note: For extra color, use different colors of green peppers.

Pork Carnitas (Instant Pot)

YIELDS: 11 SERVINGS

Nutrients: 1 net carbs ~ 20g protein ~ 7g fats ~ 160 cal.

Ingredients:

2½-lb. shoulder blade roast, trimmed and boneless

2 tsp. kosher salt

Black pepper (amount as desired)

1½ tsp. cumin

6 minced garlic cloves

½ tsp. sazon GOYA

¼ tsp. dry oregano

¾ c. reduced-sodium chicken broth

2 bay leaves

2-3 chipotle peppers in adobo sauce (to taste)

¼ tsp. dry adobo seasoning (e.g., GOYA)

½ tsp. garlic powder

How to prepare:

1. Prepare the roast with pepper and salt. Sear it for about 5 minutes in a skillet. Let it cool and insert the garlic slivers into the roast using a blade (approximately 1 inch deep). Season with the garlic powder, sazon, cumin, oregano, and adobo.

2. Arrange the chicken in the Instant Pot. Add the broth, chipotle peppers, and bay leaves. Stir and secure the lid. Prepare using high pressure for 50 minutes (meat button).
3. Naturally release the pressure and shred the pork. Combine with the juices. Discard the bay leaves.
4. Add a bit more cumin and adobo if needed. Stir well and serve.

Salsa Shredded Chicken (Instant Pot)

YIELDS: 5 SERVINGS

Nutrients: 2 net carbs ~ 22g protein ~ 3g fats ~125 cal.

Ingredients:

1 lb. chicken breast, skinless and boneless

¾ tsp. cumin

½ tsp. kosher salt

Pinch oregano

Black pepper (to taste)

1 c. chunky salsa (homemade or favorite keto version)

How to prepare:

1. Sprinkle the chicken with the spices. Add to the Instant Pot.
2. Cover with the salsa and close the lid. Set for 20 minutes. Use the natural or quick release method to remove the steam.
3. Add the chicken to a platter and shred. Serve.

Stuffed Meatloaf

YIELDS: 8 SERVINGS

Nutrients: 1.42 net carbs ~ 15.8g protein ~ 19.56g fats ~ 248.6 cal.

Ingredients:

6 slices cheddar cheese

1.65 oz. ground beef

¼ c. each:

Spinach

Mushrooms

Green onions

Yellow onions

To your liking:

Cumin

Garlic

Salt

Pepper

How to prepare:

1. Warm up the oven to 350°F.
2. Combine the meat with the garlic and spices to your liking.
3. Grease a meatloaf pan. Leave the center open for the stuffing.
4. Chop the onions. Combine with the mushrooms and spinach.

5. Mix a small amount of the beef over the top and a layer of spinach and mushrooms (for the top).

6. Bake for 1 hour and enjoy.

Slow-Cooked Venison Roast

YIELDS: 6 SERVINGS

Nutrients: 10 net carbs ~48g protein ~ 8g fats ~ 314 cal.

Ingredients:

1 boneless (3 lb.) venison roast

¼ tsp. ground black pepper

1 tbsp. each:

Worcestershire sauce

Soy sauce

Garlic salt

1 large sliced onion

1 pkg. dry onion soup mix (1 oz.)

1 can condensed cream of mushroom soup (10.75 oz.)

How to prepare:

1. Arrange the cleaned roast in the Crock-Pot and toss in the onion.
2. Drizzle with the soy sauce, Worcestershire sauce, pepper, and garlic salt.
3. Combine the soup and the pouch of soup mix. Empty it over the meat.
4. Secure the lid. Slow cook for 6 hours on low.
5. Enjoy with your favorite side dish.

Thai Green Chicken Curry (Instant Pot)

YIELDS: 6 SERVINGS

Nutrients: 5 net carbs ~ 17g protein ~ 15g fats ~ 231 cal.

Ingredients:

1 lb. chicken thighs, skinless and boneless

2 tbsp. curry paste

1 tbsp. each:

Coconut oil

Minced garlic

Minced ginger

½ c. each:

Sliced onion

Basil leaves

2 c. peeled and chopped eggplant

1 chopped yellow, green, or orange pepper

1 c. unsweetened coconut milk

2 tbsp. each:

Splenda/another sweetener

Soy sauce/coconut aminos

1 tbsp. each:

Salt

Fish sauce

How to prepare:

1. Set the Instant Pot on the Sauté function. When hot, add the oil and curry paste. Sauté for 1 to 2 minutes.
2. Toss in the garlic and ginger. Sauté about 30 seconds. Stir in the onions along with the rest of the fixings. Deglaze the pan.
3. Switch to the slow cooker mode for 8 hours using the medium setting.
4. Stir and enjoy!

Chapter 10: Special Desserts

Chocolate-Dipped Apricots

YIELDS: 36 SERVINGS

Nutrients: 4 net carbs ~ 0g protein ~ 1g fats ~ 21 cal.

Ingredients:

36 dried apricots

½ c. bittersweet chocolate chips

2 tbsp. chopped pistachios

How to prepare:

1. Prep a cookie tin with wax or parchment paper.
2. Dump the chips into a container. Microwave for a minute on medium. Stir and continue until melted (20-second intervals).
3. Dip each apricot half into the chocolate and arrange the fruit on the cookie sheet. Drizzle with the pistachios. Refrigerate for 30 minutes or until the chocolate has set.
4. Enjoy any time.

Chocolate Swirl Cheesecake Bites

YIELDS: 11 SERVINGS

Nutrients: 3.3 net carbs ~ 1.0g protein ~ 4.4g fats ~ 29.8 cal.

Ingredients:

½ tsp. vanilla extract

¼ c. + 1 tbsp. fat-free cream cheese

1 c. light whipped topping

1 tbsp. each:

Splenda

Unsweetened cocoa powder

Mini chocolate chips

How to prepare:

1. Add the cream cheese, whipped topping, vanilla, and Splenda into a mixing container. Use a mixer or fork to blend the ingredients. Add the cocoa powder and mix well.
2. Create the swirls: Add the cocoa to ½ of the batter, mix, and recombine swirling.
3. Spoon into an ice-cube tray. Top each with 5-10 mini chips.
4. Freeze for a couple of hours. Pop them out when you want a small tasty treat after dinner or any time.

Coconut Almond Cake (Instant Pot)

YIELDS: 8 SERVINGS

Nutrients: 3 net carbs ~ 5g protein ~ 23g fats ~ 236 cal.

Dry ingredients:

1 c. almond flour

½ c. unsweetened shredded coconut

⅓ c. Truvia

1 tsp. each:

Apple pie spice

Baking powder

Wet ingredients:

¼ c. melted butter

2 lightly whisked eggs

½ c. heavy whipping cream

Also needed:

1 (6-inch) round cake pan

2 c. water

How to prepare:

1. Combine all the dry fixings. Add each of the wet ingredients, one at a time.
2. Empty the batter into the pan and cover with foil.

3. Empty the water into the Instant Pot and place the steamer rack.

4. Set the timer for 40 minutes using the high-pressure setting. Naturally release for 10 minutes, then quick release.

5. Remove the pan and let it cool 15-20 minutes. Flip it over onto a platter. Garnish as desired (count the carbs).

Sugar-Free Brownies

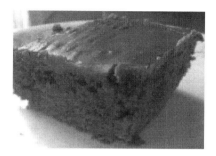

YIELDS: 25 SERVINGS

Nutrients: 4.5 net carbs ~ 1.9g protein ~ 5.7g fats ~ 74 cal.

Ingredients:

¼ c. cocoa powder, unsweetened

½ c. margarine

2 eggs

1 c. each:

All-purpose flour

Granular sucralose sweetener (Splenda)

¼ c. skim milk

⅛ tsp. salt

Optional: ½ c. chopped walnuts

Ingredients for the frosting:

1 pkg. chocolate-fudge-flavored instant pudding (1.4 oz. sugar-free)

1 c. skim milk

Also needed: 1 8-inch pan

How to prepare:

1. Program the oven to 350°F. Grease and flour the pan.
2. Use medium heat to melt the margarine and cocoa in a small saucepan. Stir periodically until smooth. Take from the heat and let it cool.
3. Beat the eggs until frothy in another bowl. Stir in the sweetener.
4. Mix the salt and flour. Blend into the egg mixture. Stir in with the margarine/cocoa mixture. Pour in the milk (¼ cup) and nuts if using.
5. Dump into the pan. Bake for approximately 25-30 minutes.
6. Prepare the frosting: Combine the pudding mix and the cup of skim milk. Blend about 2 minutes and spread over the tasty brownies. Yummy!

Conclusion

I HOPE YOU ENJOYED reading your copy of *Intermittent Fasting For Women: Powerful Strategies To Burn Fat & Lose Weight Rapidly, Control Hunger, Slow The Aging Process, & Live A Healthy Life As You Keep Your Hormones In Balance.* You should now have a better understanding of the wide variety of options available when it comes to intermittent fasting and how you can best mix and match these options to find the perfect solution for you. The decision to alter your original eating patterns is a major one, and it is crucial that you take the full weight of the decision into account before acting.

If you are convinced that you have what it takes to fully enjoy the benefits that intermittent fasting offers, the next step is to stop reading and to start fasting. Choose the type of intermittent fasting technique that seems like the best fit for you and give it a try. To begin the program, you have an abundant supply of recipes to use.

Don't become discouraged if you don't see immediate results. Try to find the plan that's right for you. Above all, don't rush. Remember that intermittent fasting is a marathon, not a sprint. Slow and steady will win the race.

The next step is to head out to the supermarket and stock up on all the goodies you'll need to begin your new lifestyle. Keep a tally of your intake and read those labels to ensure you remain within the appropriate levels for maintaining your chosen fasting method. These are some of the lessons from which you'll benefit:

- Ideally, fast 12-16 hours and fast two or three days non-consecutively; e.g., Tuesday, Thursday, and Saturday.
- Do only light cardio or yoga on your fasting days. Perform more intense workouts on non-fasting days.
- Drink plenty of liquids, including coffee and tea (no sweeteners or milk added).
- Take a two-week break and another day of fasting to your routine.

Remember, much more research is being conducted on intermittent fasting and its benefits. I hope you have gained a ton of useful information to guide you along your healthier path. Please enjoy each phase because it does work!

Finally, if you found this book useful in any way, a review on your favorite online bookstore is always appreciated!